COMPOUND SOLUTIONS

COMPOUND SOLUTIONS

Pharmaceutical Alternatives for Global Health

Susan Craddock

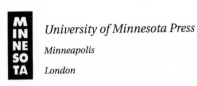

University of Minnesota Press

Minneapolis

London

Published by the University of Minnesota Press
111 Third Avenue South, Suite 290
Minneapolis, MN 55401-2520
http://www.upress.umn.edu

Printed in the United States of America on acid-free paper

The University of Minnesota is an equal-opportunity educator and employer.

23 22 21 20 19 18 17   10 9 8 7 6 5 4 3 2 1

Library of Congress Cataloging-in-Publication Data
Names: Craddock, Susan, author. | University of Minnesota Press.
Title: Compound solutions : pharmaceutical alternatives for global health / Susan Craddock.
Description: Minneapolis : University of Minnesota Press, [2017] | Includes bibliographical
    references and index.
Identifiers: LCCN 2016038249 (print) | ISBN 978-1-5179-0078-6 (hc) | ISBN 978-1-5179-0079-3 (pb)
Subjects: | MESH: Technology, Pharmaceutical | Antitubercular Agents | Global Health | Drug
    Discovery | Tuberculosis—drug therapy | Public—Private Sector Partnerships
Classification: LCC RM300 (print) | NLM QV 778 | DDC 615.1—dc23
LC record available at https://lccn.loc.gov/2016038249

To my mother
Norma Jean Craddock
1933–2008
my foundation and my inspiration

CONTENTS

ABBREVIATIONS

ARV   antiretroviral, drugs for treating AIDS
BCG   bacille Calmette-Guérin, tuberculosis vaccine
BMGF   Bill and Melinda Gates Foundation
CAB   community advisory boards, liaisons between researchers and community members for clinical trials
CSIR   Council of Scientific and Industrial Research, India: a government consortium of thirty-seven scientific laboratories
CSR   corporate social responsibility
DDW   Drugs for the Developing World, a GSK-run unit dedicated to research of infectious diseases (including tuberculosis) and located in Tres Cantos, Spain
DOTS   Directly Observed Therapy, Short-course, a method for ensuring higher regimen adherence rates by having health care workers watch patients take TB medications
EDCTP   European and Developing Countries Clinical Trials Partnership, an organization based in Europe and Africa that funds clinical trials in low-income countries
EMA   European Medicines Agency
FDA   Food and Drug Administration, the main regulatory body in the United States in charge of overseeing safety and efficacy of new drugs and vaccines and approving them for market
FDC   fixed-dose combination, multidrug regimens that are combined into one pill for greater ease of adherence
GAVI   Gavi, the Vaccine Alliance, formerly the Global Alliance for Vaccine and Immunization, a public–private organization

with the mission of getting underused and new vaccines to as many children as possible in the poorest countries

GCP   good clinical practices, part of the ICH standardization of drug research and manufacturing requirements

GSK   GlaxoSmithKline, a major UK-based pharmaceutical company

ICH   International Conference on Harmonization (1990), where rules of safety and ethics on pharmaceutical research and manufacturing were implemented. These standards are required by the FDA and EMA for approval of new drugs and vaccines.

IP   intellectual property, designating the proprietary practices of pharmaceutical companies or PDPs. Patents are IP, and PDPs have used their patents very differently from the commercial sector.

MDGs   millennium development goals

MDR-TB   multidrug-resistant tuberculosis

MSF   Médecins Sans Frontières, or Doctors Without Borders, a medical organization ministering to health emergencies in low-income regions, often among populations uprooted by war or civil strife or neglected by their governments

NIH   National Institutes of Health, an agglomeration of federally funded institutes dedicated to funding biomedical research

NSF   National Science Foundation, a federally funded organization dedicated to funding research in the sciences and social sciences

OSDD   Open Source Drug Discovery Programme, funded by the CSIR in India and focusing on research and discovery of novel therapies for diseases, including tuberculosis

PDP   product development partnership

RCT   randomized, controlled trial: the structure of clinical trial, introduced in the 1940s, aimed to eliminate bias in medical research. Participants are recruited through a randomized mechanism, then randomly divided into either the control arm (which takes the established therapy or a placebo) and the experimental arm (taking the therapy being tested).

SATVI   South African Tuberculosis Vaccine Initiative, based in Cape Town, South Africa, and part of the University of Cape Town

TAG	Treatment Action Group
TB Alliance	Global Alliance for Tuberculosis Drug Development
TBVI	Tuberculosis Vaccine Initiative, a Dutch-based vaccine research and development nonprofit company
UNICEF	United Nations Children's Fund, addresses the welfare of children in health and immunization and helps countries procure vaccines for infant and child immunization programs
WHO	World Health Organization
WIPO	World Intellectual Property Organization

LEADERS OF PRODUCT DEVELOPMENT PARTNERSHIPS, 2015

DEREK AMBROSINO, former communications manager, Global Alliance for Tuberculosis Drug Development

DAVID BARROS-AGUIRRE, director of GlaxoSmithKline's Drugs for the Developing World facility for research and development of tuberculosis drugs

JIM CONNOLLY, former president and CEO, Aeras

THOMAS EVANS, acting chief scientific officer, Aeras

DANIEL EVERITT, vice president and senior medical officer, Global Alliance for Tuberculosis Drug Development

ELIZABETH GARDINER, former vice president, market access, Global Alliance for Tuberculosis Drug Development

ANN GINSBERG, chief medical officer, Aeras; former chief medical officer at Global Alliance for Tuberculosis Drug Development; former director of project management at Merck and Company

DAVID McCOWN, senior manager, project management, Aeras

HELEN McSHANE, professor, Oxford University, and developer of TB vaccine MVA85A

CARL NATHAN, prominent tuberculosis researcher and chair of the Department of Microbiology and Immunology at the Weill Cornell Medical College, Cornell University

MEL SPIGELMAN, president and chief executive officer, Global Alliance for Tuberculosis Drug Development

DANIE THERON, superintendent of Brewelskloof, the tuberculosis hospital in Worcester, South Africa

INTRODUCTION

Changing the Paradigm of Pharmaceutical Development

As of 2014, tuberculosis has surpassed AIDS as the leading cause of death globally from an infectious disease. According to the 2015 World Health Organization (WHO) *Global Tuberculosis Report*, at least 1.5 million persons died from tuberculosis, and 9.6 million became sick with it. One million cases and 140,000 deaths were in children, and just over a million individuals coinfected with HIV were estimated to develop tuberculosis in 2014. Of these, however, only about one third were put on antiretroviral (ARV) therapy. Almost half a million new cases of multidrug-resistant tuberculosis (MDR-TB) are also estimated to have occurred in 2014, yet only one quarter of these were actually diagnosed and reported (WHO 2015).

All in all, these numbers are disheartening for a preventable bacterial disease that has had drug regimens available for decades to effectively treat it. It has proved tenacious where other entrenched infectious diseases such as smallpox and polio have been eradicated, or nearly eradicated. And though incidence rates have fallen in sixteen out of the twenty-two highest-burden countries that account for around 80 percent of all tuberculosis cases, this reduction has been minor in most cases and very slow. In the rest of the high-burden countries, incidence rates have hit a plateau or continue to rise (WHO 2015).

This last sentence holds the key to tuberculosis's tenacity, as well as to the subject of this book. Though technically caused by the bacterium *Mycobacterium tuberculosis*, tuberculosis does not occur evenly across geographic and social boundaries. It thrives in those parts of the world where poverty in all its forms of structural violence including crowding, the retrenchment of government services, food insecurity, underemployment, discrimination, low wages, and inadequate access to health care or effective drugs and diagnostics maintain a stronghold. Those twenty-two countries burdened with high levels of tuberculosis are the same countries appearing at the bottom of other indices developed by global institutions like the WHO or the World Bank to measure quality of life and economy. Within countries, tuberculosis is found concentrated in the poorest regions and neighborhoods, a predictable testament to the interrelation of deprivation and disease. Global statistics, then, are misleading given the huge discrepancies in tuberculosis rates between richer and poorer countries, and between well-resourced and impoverished regions within countries. South Africa's rate of new tuberculosis cases, for example, is 834/100,000, while in the United States it is 3/100,000 (WHO 2015). And individuals living in KwaZulu-Natal, one of the poorest provinces in South Africa, were more than twice as likely to die of tuberculosis in 2009 as their counterparts in wealthier provinces of the country (UNDP 2009). As Gerry Kearns and Simon Reid-Henry note in their article on vital geographies (2009), despite so many advances in technology and medical research, where you are born in the world remains starkly determinant of how well, and how long, you are likely to live.

The persistence of tuberculosis can be attributed to many factors in addition to the persistence of poverty: the failure of previous mitigation efforts, the tenacity of the bacillus that causes tuberculosis, inequitable global economies, and during the last decades of the twentieth century, the unwillingness of global organizations and governments to address it. In effect, Western governments turned their attention away from tuberculosis in the mid-twentieth century after the advent of antibiotics and improved economies contributed to its dramatic decline from all but the poorest and most invisible sectors of their populations. By the 1970s, even the WHO stopped treating tuberculosis as a high priority, subsuming national tuberculosis programs into larger respiratory or communicable disease departments and cutting support for TB experts (Raviglione and Pio 2002).

A resurgence of tuberculosis in the United States and Europe in the 1980s and high rates of HIV/TB coinfection in many countries put tuberculosis back on the map. Funding to combat it, however, remains disproportionately low relative to the number of people it effects: the Global Fund to Fight AIDS, TB, and Malaria, for example, allocated more than 50 percent of its budget to fight AIDS, and only 16 percent for tuberculosis (2015). The bacille Calmette-Guérin, or BCG vaccine, invented almost a century ago has proven minimal in its protection of adolescents and adults, and the current drug regimen, developed decades ago, takes six to nine months for patients to complete. Despite this dismal situation and the devastating toll it is taking, the pharmaceutical industry has turned a blind eye to this situation given the lack of financial incentive inherent in the poverty of tuberculosis sufferers. It is not surprising, then, that South Africa's minister of health, Aaron Motsoaledi, bemoaned recently at an international lung health conference that "tuberculosis is the disease that has killed the most people in the last two hundred years: more than smallpox, malaria, plague, and influenza. Yet it is still not considered a serious crisis" (2014).

It is in this context of widespread suffering but limited attention that two nonprofit collaborations, the Global Alliance for Tuberculosis Drug Development, or TB Alliance, and Aeras, have formed with the specific purpose of developing new drugs and vaccines for tuberculosis for the first time in over forty years. Part of a new emphasis in global health initiatives called product development partnerships (PDPs), TB Alliance and Aeras partner with university researchers, government and philanthropic donors, biotech and pharmaceutical companies, and global public health agencies like the WHO to come up with vaccines that are more effective in reducing disease and transmission as well as drug regimens that work faster and can combat MDR-TB and HIV coinfection. Their goal is to drastically reduce the number of new infections and to eventually achieve zero deaths from tuberculosis through the development of these new biotechnologies. How they are going about achieving this goal is the main focus of this book.

The mission of both PDPs is to produce drug regimens and vaccines that are accessible, affordable, and available to all who need them. Yet producing new pharmaceuticals is an enormously expensive enterprise, and one where corners cannot be cut to reduce costs. Developing low-cost therapies for millions of poor individuals, therefore, is an especially challenging and even contradictory endeavor. Accordingly, TB Alliance and Aeras are forging new and innovative approaches to therapeutic research and development at the same time they are developing the therapies themselves. They are engaging in what I am calling humanitarian pharmaceutical production. The therapies they produce are neither commercial nor generic. They are an entirely different product from their commercial counterparts.

To elaborate, commercial pharmaceuticals today are highly geared toward markets: what therapies get developed typically are what will earn the highest profits, not what will help the most people. This bottom line does not preclude the development of lifesaving vaccines and drugs when this matches up with a sufficient, and sufficiently financed, consumer base: the hypertension, diabetes, and cancer drugs developed in recent years are powerful testament to that. It is thus not inaccurate to state, as one large pharmaceutical company does on its website, that they "want to help people to do more, feel better, live longer" (www.gsk.com).

The question is, who do they make feel better and live longer? The London and New York Stock Exchange share prices listed on the same web page for their investors and "updated every 15 and 20 minutes respectively" are a clue to answering that question. Most major pharmaceutical companies today are publicly traded, which means they are beholden first and foremost to their shareholders and thus to a minimum threshold return on dollars invested. Consumers in higher-income countries who have sufficient insurance or incomes to "pay what the market can bear" for drugs are the ones the pharmaceutical industry is making feel better and live longer—not the poor in low-income countries. Pharmaceuticals have become key determinants of the geographic coordinates of inequality in twenty-first-century capitalism, but also of the increasing alienation of the world's poor from resources such as medicines necessary to well-being.

TB Alliance and Aeras on the other hand are asking a very different set of questions about why pharmaceutical development should happen, how, and for whom. They are proposing to turn pharmaceuticals into critical components ameliorating the lives and well-being of the world's impoverished rather than the opposite. They are seeing pharmaceuticals as first and foremost technologies for keeping people alive, rather than tools of profit generation. In this, TB Alliance and Aeras follow in the wake of a global alliance of AIDS activists who campaigned in the late 1990s and early 2000s to reduce the costs of highly active ARV therapy so that those living with AIDS in poor countries could access these lifesaving medicines like their counterparts in rich countries. The brutal contradiction of millions dying from AIDS each year while effective but expensive drugs existed transformed access to drugs from a public health to a human rights issue (Heywood 2002; Messac and Prabhu 2013; Mbali 2013). Aeras and TB Alliance do not specifically employ the language of human rights in the work that they do, yet they employ in their fundamental philosophy and practices the motto of the AIDS campaign, putting "people before profits." Their endeavors are humanitarian by virtue of tethering pharmaceutical production to global health need, and in particular by striving to get new technologies out and into the bodies of millions of people with, or at risk of, tuberculosis no matter how poor they are.

The main argument animating the rest of this book is that PDPs' innovations extend well beyond the products they are developing. The humanitarian mooring of their endeavors means both an expansion and an alteration of the social, political, logistical, and scientific fields pharmaceutical developers typically occupy or that pharmaceuticals occupy (Petryna, Lakoff, and Kleinman 2006). TB Alliance and Aeras are thus not just developing new pharmaceuticals as we have come to understand that term. The philosophies, individuals, and relations they encompass and that constitute them are in turn redefining them. New tuberculosis therapies *are* the politics and finances, poverty and promises they are confronting. They are entanglements—inextricable interrelations—of scientific endeavors, regulatory policies, the nature of the bacillus, community desires, disease burdens, and government–institutional relations, to name a few, that make them necessary and possible. They possess multivalent meanings, representing hope to potential consumers, logistical challenges to government or regulatory authorities, better tools for medical practitioners, and increased opportunities for scientists in high-burden countries. Their value comes from the multiple spheres of social, political, and economic capital they create: in the possibility of keeping millions alive, thereby restoring human capital; in signaling by default the economic and political conditions sustaining widespread vulnerability to tuberculosis; by working against predominant relations of pharmaceutical production; and by saving millions of dollars in costs of hospitalization and diminished labor productivity. PDPs in other words are forcing a shift in the ontological mooring of today's market-driven neoliberal pharmaceutical industry.

A further question then becomes whether a more humanitarian model of pharmaceuticals production is capable of reconfiguring the incentives and structures of mainstream pharmaceutical production. In Timothy Mitchell's discussion of taking account of modernity and its coordinates, he argues that alternative modes of capitalist modernity need to be included. Their incompatibility constituting them as outside the otherwise singular logic of modern, Western, capitalist formations, these alternative movements according to Mitchell are critical for how they

"continually redirect, divert, and mutate the modernity they help constitute" (2000, xiii). Tuberculosis PDPs continuously negotiate the exact
terms of their alterity as they strive to realize their mission. Yet they also
contend with research and development processes that are expensive
and time consuming, and with partners in academia, philanthropy, or
industry who have divergent motivations for participating in humanitarian pharmaceutical endeavors. TB Alliance and Aeras thus highlight the
necessity and distinct possibilities, but also challenges, of incorporating
alternative logics into contemporary (post)modern capitalist formations
within the pharmaceutical sector.

Because they are forging new relations of therapeutic development,
PDPs do not operate with specific blueprints, but have a degree of latitude for innovation and for creating different kinds of partnerships that
fit the particular products they are developing. The basic symbiosis of
nonprofit and industry collaboration was made abundantly clear to me
by numerous informants. Those from the nonprofit sector pointed to
pharmaceutical company resources including money, laboratory facilities, and vast chemical libraries,[1] plus the enhanced ability of private
industry to attract scientists across the biomedical, clinical, and pharmacological disciplines necessary for chemotherapeutic development.
Those from industry readily admit the invaluable role nonprofit agencies
play in pipeline development, community outreach, ascertaining regional
variations in technology adoption, and discussing regulatory approvals
or purchasing and distribution plans with the WHO and other purchasing
entities and relevant governments.

Equally important to how PDPs function are a range of factors including the tuberculosis bacterium itself, regulatory structures, funding priorities, political environments, laboratory and clinical facilities, and
current limits to scientific knowledge. As this book will make clear, the
tenacity of the tuberculosis bacterium and inadequate understanding of
the immune system are critically important in shaping what is possible
in new drug and vaccine development. Taken together, these networks
are not just responding to particular realities or solutions, but rather are
dynamically creating new realities as they play out (Mol 2002). As Aihwa
Ong suggests, assemblages or networks of new biotechnological production do not necessarily follow "given scales or political mappings," but
create their own spaces and give new meanings to the actors and practices involved (2005, 338).

There are significant challenges that PDPs face, however. Tuberculosis needs not just one but a regimen of drugs with differing mechanisms of action—that is, different ways drugs act on the bacterium in the body—to successfully rid the body of infection. Coupled with generally low success rates of new drug or vaccine candidates in the pharmaceutical development pipelines, typically 10 percent, even several new candidates suddenly become deeply inadequate despite representing a significant improvement over no new candidates a decade ago. This contradiction of so much more than before, yet still so inadequate, signals the precariousness that comes along with the promise of PDPs. Much of this precariousness, ironically, is the flip side of innovative models of pharmaceuticals development. Disassociating drug and vaccine production from profit incentives brings many advantages in terms of the potential to address public health needs, but it also brings the greatest challenge at least in the shorter term as PDPs face the prohibitive expenses of compound research and development.

The reasons for these expenses are multiple. Drugs and vaccines take years to develop, going from preclinical discovery phases all the way through three phases of clinical (human) testing and regulatory approval. Discovery phases include creating new compounds in the laboratory and screening existing compounds for efficacy against *M. tuberculosis*, while in the preclinical phase promising compounds are tested for safety and toxicity in animals. Clinical phases include Phase I trials conducted in a very small number of usually healthy individuals to further determine early signs of efficacy, safety, side effects, and metabolism of the new drug or vaccine in humans. Phase IIa and IIb trials involve testing a compound for efficacy, correct dosing, and immunogenicity among a larger number of individuals with the condition (such as tuberculosis) in the case of drug trials or who are vulnerable to the condition in the case of vaccine trials. Finally, Phase III trials gather further evidence of efficacy and proper dosing either alone or against existing drugs or vaccines and are conducted typically across numerous sites and countries in tens of thousands of individuals. Because of their size and complexity, Phase III trials are prohibitively expensive and contribute to a significant portion of the estimated $2 billion that it will cost to license a TB vaccine and the $5 billion to generate adequate new TB drugs, according to the WHO's Stop TB Partnership (n.d.).

An elaboration is useful here of why new therapies are needed if there is already a vaccine and effective drugs for tuberculosis. The BCG vaccine for tuberculosis works to prevent pulmonary tuberculosis (TB of the lungs) in infants, but the protection is inadequate and it wears off by later childhood. Adults and adolescents are not protected at all. Though the BCG is still in wide use, it is widely acknowledged that a much better vaccine is needed for prevention of infection or prevention of disease. Vaccines also need to be found for those coinfected with HIV, since the BCG is not recommended for infants with HIV or for anyone with compromised immune systems.

Currently the regimen recommended by the Centers for Disease Control and Prevention and WHO for drug-susceptible tuberculosis consists of an initial phase of two months on all four of the drugs considered to be "first line," or standard regimen, that is, isoniazid (INH), rifampicin (RIF), ethambutol (EMB), and pyrazinamide (PZA). After completing the designated number of doses of these four medications, the patient is pared down to just isoniazid and rifampicin for another four to seven months (CDC 2010; WHO 2009). The most evident problems with this regimen are the length of time it takes to complete, the corresponding difficulty individuals can have in taking multiple drugs over six to nine months when potable water might not always be available, and when symptoms improve early on and patients assume they no longer need to stay on the regimen. Though Directly Observed Therapy, Short-course (DOTS), where health-care workers supervise patients taking their medications, has been utilized to good effect to improve adherence in many areas, it is expensive and difficult for low-income governments to maintain over time (TB Alliance 2000). If drug-susceptible patients do manage to stay on their regimens, current first-line drugs remain 95 percent effective. Yet problems are not limited to enduring a lengthy therapeutic process. Adverse drug reactions prevent those significant numbers coinfected with HIV and taking ARV therapy from taking first-line TB drugs; and dosing for children with tuberculosis is difficult since these drugs are only now being tested in this population (Lessem 2014a).

Length of current treatment is also a critical factor in the rapidly rising rate of MDR-TB. Indeed the rise of MDR-TB has generated even greater impetus to, and urgency for, developing drugs with new methods for combating the bacterium, as well as shorter treatment regimens. Drug resistance happens for several reasons, only one of them being poor adherence. Other reasons include inferior drug quality, inadequate dosing, monotherapy (taking only one drug instead of a full regimen), or inappropriate drug regimens (Chen-Yuan 2010). Increasingly, however, MDR-TB is also a result of direct transmission. Though it has existed for decades, available evidence suggests that MDR-TB is on the rise across many regions of the world: by 2007, systematic surveys found MDR-TB in eighty-two countries and drug-resistant strains in ninety (Mitnick et al. 2007). In some regions its rise appears precipitous, with for example an estimated 20 percent of all new TB cases now multidrug resistant in eastern Europe (TB Alliance 2013). In many regions diagnosis of MDR-TB is low, with China for example having only an estimated 11 percent of its MDR-TB cases diagnosed. Poor diagnosis and treatment of MDR-TB in turn is leading to a rise in extensively drug-resistant tuberculosis, or XDR-TB. It is now reported in 105 countries with an estimated 9.7 percent of MDR-TB cases reclassified as XDR-TB (WHO 2015).

Even with MDR-TB, the poor are especially vulnerable. As one recent editorial by Salman Keshavjee and Paul Farmer suggests, "from New York City to Karachi to Maseru" poor populations including the homeless, migrants, immunocompromised, and malnourished are not just more vulnerable to drug-susceptible tuberculosis. Poverty also fuels higher rates of MDR-TB through overcrowding (whether in prisons or in homes) as do limited access to quality health care capable of accurate and prompt diagnosis, sustained access to quality-assured drugs, and effective means of therapeutic delivery (Keshavjee and Farmer 2010, 1222). It is not, then, that MDR-TB is incurable. Evidence from various regions suggests that relatively high treatment success rates of 60 to 70 percent or higher are possible with careful management of MDR-TB patients (Caminero 2010; Kuaban 2011). The problem is that these rates are too rarely achieved.

One reason, as implied above, has to do with the nature of the drugs themselves. Evidence varies about the minimum number of drugs MDR-TB patients should take to ensure effective treatment, but a relatively standard number is five. Five different antibiotics means typically around twenty pills and one injection every day for eighteen to twenty-four months (Brigden 2011). Many discussions I heard among clinicians during MDR-TB sessions at tuberculosis conferences revolved around how to manage the many and sometimes severe side effects of these drugs. They focused as well on how to keep patients on their regimens for the duration given the difficulties in doing so and given the impact on their bodies and their morale. As one public health official from Indonesia commented at a 2011 conference, many MDR-TB patients are as much in need of psychological counseling as of drug treatment given the emotional burden of treatment as well as diagnosis (Aditama 2011).

In addition to their complexity, length of time to complete, inadequacy, and toxicity, second-line drugs are expensive. This fact indicates why patents are not the only factor determining the price of drugs, since patents have long since expired on all second-line tuberculosis drugs. The reason for high costs is that most of these drugs have only one producer given the lack of incentive to manufacture drugs for limited, low-income populations (MSF 2009). Pharmaceutical companies often have an internal mandate to continue producing a drug if there is medical need and they are the only ones left producing it (Gail Cassell, former vice president of scientific affairs, Eli Lilly, personal communication, March 17, 2009), but low-volume production with no competition typically means higher prices. As a result, second-line tuberculosis drugs cost $1,800 to $7,300 and more per patient for a two-year regimen (MSF 2009).

Not only can very few patients afford those prices, many resource-limited countries cannot or will not pay for second-line TB drugs when other critical health problems affecting larger populations claim higher priority. One manufacturer also means frequent interruptions of supply, sometimes worldwide (Caminero 2010), as well as inadequate supplies to meet demand. In 2011, for example, there was a global shortage of capreomycin, a key injectable drug for treating MDR-TB patients. Akorn, the only quality-assured manufacturer of capreomycin, could not get the active pharmaceutical ingredient for producing the drug. In 2010, there was another worldwide shortage of a critical drug for MDR-TB treatment, kanamycin. The result of these shortages is the inability of MDR-TB patients to complete or start their drug regimens, exacerbating burdens of suffering and increasing the likelihood of death (Brigden 2011). Together, these reasons form a compelling case for new tuberculosis therapies, and for forming the collaborations needed to develop them.

Collaborations and the Changing Terrain of Patents

Collaboration especially between the pharmaceutical industry and research universities is not new. What is new about PDPs today is why they form collaborations and for what kinds of pharmaceutical products. Why collaborations are needed to produce pharmaceuticals for diseases like tuberculosis is linked, among other things, to developments in the pharmaceutical industry. It is only relatively recently that the pharmaceutical industry became so inextricably tied to profit incentives, in the process turning its attention to some diseases and markets to the exclusion of others. The profit motive behind pharmaceuticals production itself is not new: commercial potential understandably has been a concern of pharmaceutical companies for decades. What has changed in part is the role and regulation of patents in pharmaceuticals development. There is nothing inherent in the legal rights conferred by the award of a patent that dictates how it will be used—indeed, in answering the question of what a patent is, the U.S. Patent and Trademark Office makes clear that it does not grant the right to "make, use, offer for sale, sell or import," but rather grants the right to exclude *others* from "making, using, offering for sale, selling or importing the invention" (USPTO 2010). It grants, in other words, a proprietary right to control the use of a new discovery.

As numerous historians of medicine have pointed out, throughout much of the twentieth century patents played a highly controversial role in both industry- and university-based pharmaceuticals research (Apple 1989; Gaudillière 2008; Bud 2008; Gabriel 2014). A critical element of this controversy was the widespread notion that medicines in particular should remain in the public domain, since patenting them could threaten to derail further scientific research and therapeutic access. By the nineteenth century, France and Germany had banned patents on medicines (Bud 2008). By the 1930s many high-visibility research universities in the United States including Harvard, the University of Pennsylvania, Johns Hopkins, and Columbia either restricted or mandated against patenting of medical discoveries by their faculty. Similarly, the British Medical Research Council, Royal College of Physicians, and Royal College of Surgeons met in 1932 and called for an international treaty banning patents on medicines (Bud 2008, 178).

The next several decades nevertheless saw patents increasing on medical discoveries for a variety of reasons. Drug firms, for one thing, came to see patents as effective tools of scientific innovation rather than the opposite, when returns on patented discoveries reached levels sufficient to reinvest in further research (Slinn 2008). The advent of penicillin and sulfa drugs in the 1930s and 1940s was particularly significant as they were the first drugs capable of curing a wide range of infections, which many firms quickly realized heightened commercial potential and provided the impetus to patent subsequent antibiotics and other discoveries (Tobbell 2012; Bud 2008). Advances in chemical and biological research in Germany provided the subsequent rationale to expand interpretations of what was considered patentable in drug discovery processes (Gaudillière 2008). As Gaudillière notes, these and other factors help explain why patents in the United States and Europe went within a few decades from being resisted by a wide range of academics, health professionals, and even industry representatives to becoming "so 'natural' as to be taken for granted in contemporary medicine" (2008, 128).

Despite patents' increasing importance to the drug-discovery process and to the everyday practices of pharmaceutical companies, there was still a degree of latitude governing both the extent to which patents were utilized among firms (with firms in the United States, for example, patenting at much higher rates), as well as what function they played. As Slinn (2008), for example, discusses, the therapeutic revolution of the mid-twentieth century saw increased patenting but also numerous cross-licensing arrangements between U.S. and UK pharmaceutical firms that enabled technology transfers for further scientific developments.[2] Consequent interfirm collaborations also aided overseas marketing expansion until the 1960s, when more companies had established branches across the Atlantic (Slinn 2008). During the same period, Tobbell (2012) has compellingly described for the United States the rise of collaborations between pharmaceutical firms and university researchers. As companies like Merck vertically restructured after World War II to incorporate more research as well as marketing potential, major universities were recognized as prime sites of scientific research across relevant biomedical and pharmacological fields. Cultivating particular relationships such as industry-funded postdoctoral fellowships ensured that university scientists received training in areas relevant to drug development such as clinical pharmacology, while also ensuring sustained circulations of scientific advances between universities and pharmaceutical firms—but with pharmaceutical firms retaining the fruits of fellows' research (Tobbell 2012, 27; Quirke 2007). Finally, these very purposefully nurtured collaborative relationships between industry and university were a means of offsetting government support of biomedicine, which from the 1950s onwards in the United States concentrated on building and sustaining biomedical expertise through mechanisms such as the National Institutes of Health (NIH) and the creation of the National Science Foundation (NSF) in 1950 (Tobbell 2012, 26).

The degree to which industry–university and university–government relations within biomedical research remained separate, however, changed significantly in 1980. So, too, did the role of the patent, the focus of research, and the nature of collaborative relations. In 1980 the U.S. Congress passed the Bayh-Dole Act in response to what was widely perceived as inefficiencies in the U.S. government's ability to get drugs, vaccines, or other new biotechnologies quickly onto the market. Prior to 1980, new technologies developed by university scientists using federal funds such as grants from the NIH or NSF automatically belonged to the federal government. In turn, it was the government's responsibility to ensure the widespread dissemination of these discoveries to the public. By 1980, however, evidence appeared to indicate that federally held patents were not being adequately commercialized and that changes in patenting and licensing arrangements might amend the situation.[3] The Bayh-Dole Patent and Trademark Amendments Act of 1980, then, allowed university researchers to file for patents on any discoveries made using federal funds and to license these patents to third parties. More specifically, the act encouraged exclusive licensing of new technologies to private companies in the hopes that industry would quickly turn new discoveries into commercial products (Rai and Eisenberg 2003). Bayh-Dole was not just about expediting dissemination of beneficial new technologies to the public, then. It was also about realizing a return on taxpayers' investments, a "Congressional endorsement of the argument that failure to establish patent protection over the results of federally funded university research would limit the commercial exploitation of these results" (Mowery et al. 2001, 102). Failure to practice the option of exclusive licensing of these patents could also dissuade private firms from investing in new technologies, since conferring rights of new product manufacturing and marketing to a single company was the primary guarantee of adequate profits by eliminating competition for the duration of the patent.

Simultaneous with the Bayh-Dole Act were two other factors widely acknowledged to have significant impact on patenting and licensing arrangements. The first was the 1980 Supreme Court decision *Diamond vs. Chakrabarty* that opened the doors to expanded interpretations of what was patentable by upholding the patent eligibility of genetically engineered microorganisms previously construed as too close to what is found in nature to qualify for proprietary control. The second was the establishment in 1982 of the Court of Appeals for the Federal Circuit, the final appeals court for patent cases that subsequently displayed a track record for upholding patents in 80 percent of cases versus 30 percent before 1982 (Katz et al. 1990, quoted in Mowery et al. 2001, 103).

The convergence of these three legal and legislative initiatives has resulted in significant changes in the degree, extent, and nature of patenting. One change is a substantial increase in university patenting and licensing. Between 1969 and 1979, the number of university patents went from 188 to 264; between 1979 and 1984, the number of patents more than doubled; and they more than doubled again between 1984 and 1989—from 551 to 1,228 (Mowery et al. 2001). Between 1998 and 2008, the number of patents granted to universities ranged from 2,950 to 3,700 (NSF 2010). Second, this increase includes more "upstream" patenting on cell lines, mechanisms, early-stage research, and processes, arguably making it more difficult to conduct scientific research without patent infringement and resulting in new products sometimes having patents in multiples of ten or more. From the scientist's perspective, the proliferation of patents has advantages and disadvantages. On the one hand, increased university support for patenting and licensing enhances the likelihood that discoveries will actually reach the market. On the other hand, research can be held up because patents with broad-based research applications such as processes, delivery methods, or organisms mean scientists through their universities have to negotiate licensing fees on these patents at other universities or at biotech or pharmaceutical firms before they can utilize them in their own labs.

Third, the number of university–industry partnerships also increased (Kesselheim 2011), but these new partnerships are no longer about fostering scientific exchanges. Rather, industry is now concerned that university scientists pursue lines of research with the most potential for commercialization. University Technology Transfer Offices that have sprung up as a result of Bayh-Dole channel new and potentially lucrative discoveries through the patenting process, and subsequently negotiate exclusive licensing contracts to pharmaceutical or biotechnology firms. In return for further developing and marketing these new discoveries, firms remit usually 6–10 percent of subsequent profits to universities. In 2002, the gross revenue universities acquired through licensing arrangements was close to $1 billion (Kesselheim 2011, 460). Even in universities, then, pursuing research and discovery in areas of low financial return is less common, either because it is dissuaded by institutions seeking financial returns on their scientists' patents or because of more formal or contractual relationships with pharmaceutical companies. Where research on diseases like tuberculosis still thrives, discoveries often languish in the pipeline because there is no money to take them beyond early-stage research.

The most significant change for the purposes of this book, then, is the role patents have come to play in biotechnological research: from flexible tools facilitating further scientific discovery or preventing rampant commercialization, they have become largely entrenched as critical components of highly selective research trajectories and of profit generation.

Though there is no absolute equivalent in Europe of the Bayh-Dole Act, in 1988 the EU passed a directive on biotechnologies to "harmonize and strengthen biotech patent law" (Schroeder 2009). Seeing greater public–private coordination of scientific research as a means to strengthen economic competitiveness, the EU's directive was intended to accommodate new arenas of research, to attract more investment capital, and to more strongly link university and industry (Schroeder 2009). In other words, it was intended to have the same effect as the Bayh-Dole Act and to achieve for Europe the same acceleration of scientific production and commercialization seen in the United States.

Finally, in 1994 the World Trade Organization (WTO) passed the Trade Related Aspects of Intellectual Property (TRIPS), a sweeping directive enforcing intellectual property (IP) regulations for the first time in all WTO member states. Previous to TRIPS many countries had variable regulations concerning patents on medicines, including no or limited patents, or patents on processes but not products. TRIPS requires all countries in the WTO to recognize patents on biotechnologies including drugs and vaccines and to extend the life of a patent to twenty years. It is widely acknowledged that the United States, EU, and Japan ensured the passage of TRIPS, as it opened the way for their constituent pharmaceutical and biotechnology industries to extend product patents globally, access middle- and high-income markets in more countries, and charge high prices for technologies while eliminating generic competition. Though a few, namely pharmaceutical representatives, have maintained that patents function primarily to ensure sustained research and development resources for new drugs (see Herrling 2007), a majority of scholars conclude that patents are the key mechanism enabling and sustaining prohibitive drug prices and consequently keeping drugs from sick people (see Heywood 2002; Goozner 2005).

Contestation of TRIPS was not the unique purview of scholars, however. A majority of WTO representatives from the Global South concurred with this view of the damaging role of patents within TRIPS, namely the impact pharmaceutical patents would have to public health and to people's lives. Many of these countries were suffering huge burdens of AIDS, tuberculosis, and other infectious diseases, but it was AIDS in particular that pointed to the inestimable harm that TRIPS would do. The South African grassroots organization Treatment Action Campaign was particularly successful in making visible the devastating impact of not having access to ARVs in a country with one of the highest AIDS rates in the world (Heywood 2002). Other countries like Thailand and India, with both high rates of AIDS and pharmaceutical industries capable of manufacturing cheaper generic versions of ARVs, also made apparent the inevitable outcome of TRIPS regulations. Their collective, increasingly strident protests resulted finally in the 2001 Doha Declaration, which acknowledges the effect TRIPS likely has had and would continue to have in limiting many countries' ability to access needed medicines. It thus allowed countries to grant compulsory licenses allowing manufacture and import of patented drugs at lower prices without the consent of the patent owner (MSF 2003). The amendments incorporated into the Doha agreement, however, were sufficiently complicated to result in very few countries utilizing them (WHO 2006a).

What's in a Name: Defining Neglect

The result of these national, regional, and global regulations has been the emergence of what has come to be called neglected diseases. Neglected in this instance does not mean invisible; development reports from institutions like the World Bank and annual WHO bulletins evidence the persistent high burdens of infectious diseases in low-income regions, chronicling with various statistical instruments the staggering economic and quality-of-life impacts these diseases have on populations across the globe. Neglected, here, is a very specific term referring to the gradual closing off of development pipelines for new drugs or vaccines for these infectious diseases as pharmaceutical production increasingly has come to pivot around market potential rather than disease burden. A widely cited statistic shows that between 1975 and 2004, 1,556 new chemical entities were marketed globally, yet only twenty of these, or 1.3 percent, were for infectious diseases including tuberculosis even though these diseases accounted for 12 percent of the world's disease burden in 2007. This is despite the significant increase of resources going into biomedical innovation in recent decades—from $30 billion in 1986 to $163 billion in 2009 (MSF 2011). As pharmaceutical consultants assisting a Government Accounting Office study on new drug development reported, shareholders of pharmaceutical firms—and the largest firms including Merck, Sanofi,

Pfizer, Eli Lilly, Novartis, and GlaxoSmithKline (GSK) are all publicly traded—demand a particular profit threshold for each compound moving down the development pipeline. If a compound is not expected to make this threshold, typically $200–$500 million, it does not get developed (GAO 2006). Clearly, this leaves little room for large pharmaceutical firms to pursue new drugs or vaccines targeted for markets that cannot come close to such a threshold.

Even within the rubric of "neglected disease," however, there is political and conceptual debate. Alex Broadbent astutely notes, for example, that research and development investment is neither an adequate nor accurate way to define neglect given that "it is possible to reduce the disease burden of many of these diseases without further R&D investment, and R&D investment is not necessarily the best way to reduce the burden of these diseases" (2011, 51). That social and economic deprivation is strongly associated with high rates of tuberculosis has been known for a long time and illustrates well Broadbent's point. Reducing burdens of poverty, improving nutrition, and ensuring minimum standards of housing are known to be critical components in mitigating tuberculosis transmission, as evidenced by McKeown's now classic study published in 1979.[4] Yet redressing economic and social deprivations can be difficult at best in underresourced areas, whether for ameliorating tuberculosis or other infectious disease burdens. As numerous studies have recently shown, increased privatization, market fundamentalism, and austerity measures such as state welfare retrenchment in many areas of the world have resulted in increased poverty levels and economic inequality. They have also often resulted in new fees on health care, underresourced health-care systems, too few physicians, nurses, and clinical facilities, and facilities that are inconsistently stocked with drugs or diagnostics. These, in turn, negatively impact disease burdens (see Schrecker et al. 2010 for an overview).

The fact that preventive measures against tuberculosis have long since largely been implemented in some areas of the world but not others brings us back to Broadbent's ultimate definition of neglected diseases, which takes into account not only the extent of a disease burden, but the inequities of global economic systems. According to Broadbent, ultimately "a disease D is neglected to the extent that it poses a significant health burden on some reasonably large population, and preventive, curative, or mitigatory measures are either widespread among other populations, or would be much more actively sought if D imposed a similar burden on other populations" (2011, 54). This definition is commendable because it gets beyond a mere technical or financial calculus of neglect to encompass the moral politics behind whether and what kind of interventions, including pharmaceutical, are mobilized for which populations.

On the one hand, global agencies such as the United Nations and the WHO pass resolutions to address the diseases of poverty and create mechanisms to finance interventions, one example being the 2002 Global Fund to Fight AIDS, Tuberculosis, and Malaria. Yet on the other hand are high-level WTO meetings in which inequitable terms of trade and patent protections are regularly negotiated by wealthy countries such as the United States to the detriment of lower-income regions. Many of the trade policies emerging from these meetings contribute to the very diseases the WHO is trying to fight because they often increase poverty, food insecurity, and drug prices and because they make it more difficult for many nonindustrial countries to earn currency through exports given U.S. and EU subsidies, especially of their agricultural sectors (Labonte 2001). Working in the silos that they do, then, means UN and other global agencies end up with policies, treaties, and regulations functioning at cross-purposes. It also means by extension that producing new biotechnologies within these conflicting terms can result in populations in wealthier countries gaining access while those in poorer countries do not (Sunder Rajan 2006; Ong 2010; Jasanoff 2006).

Tuberculosis is actually not considered a neglected disease by two major arbiters of such designations, namely the WHO and Médecins Sans Frontières (MSF; Doctors Without Borders). Largely this is because tuberculosis receives far more attention and funding than many infectious diseases including Chagas' disease, leishmaniasis, or schistosomiasis. As with most battles emerging from the reality of scarce resources, scarcity itself becomes a relative as well as contested term. Tuberculosis is part of the Global Fund to Fight Tuberculosis, AIDS, and Malaria, thus achieving a level of visibility and support that many infectious diseases have not attained and are not likely to. Variations in degree of neglect have thus led to designations among some scholars and agencies of "very neglected" versus "neglected" diseases (Chaudhuri 2010). I argue that tuberculosis does fit Broadbent's definition of neglect because some parts of the world largely have been able to eliminate the disease through social and economic measures as well as better drug access, because tuberculosis continues to cause huge burdens of disease across much of the world, and because a better vaccine and more and better drugs potentially could make a significant difference to the disease burden. Continuing the theme of relative neglect, tuberculosis received around 2 percent of total U.S. development assistance for health, while HIV/AIDS received over 36 percent of total funding (Liese, Rosenberg, and Schratz 2010). Even the designation of tuberculosis by the United States as a security issue has not had significant impact on funding. While such a designation in current post-9/11 politics typically mobilizes more resources for research, other infectious diseases such as anthrax or smallpox are higher up the list of security concerns. As one former tuberculosis nonprofit representative expressed to me in frustration, "what is it about two million deaths a year that doesn't warrant funding?" (Peg Willingham, former senior director of external affairs, Aeras, personal communication, June 16, 2010).

Global Health, PDPs, and the Reembrace of Technology

The development of neglected diseases did not lead inexorably to the emergence of PDPs, however. That came as a result of institutions within the larger field of global health turning their collective attention toward persistent diseases of the Global South and toward mechanisms that could mobilize private and public sector strengths in combating them. A convergence of recent historical, economic, and institutional factors deserves further elaboration for why the turn to tuberculosis, and why PDPs, at this particular moment in time.

As more than one scholar has noted (e.g., Koplan et al. 2009; Farmer, Kleinman, and Basilico 2013; Biehl and Petryna 2014), the field of global health is one that is difficult to pin down as to what exactly it is: what makes it different from the field of international health that preceded it, what its motives and shared ideologies might be, or which health issues constitute the objects of its attention. International health was marked by state-sponsored initiatives coordinated by global organizations such as the WHO, often with an unreflective assumption that Western expertise would be critical to reducing disease burdens in colonial or newly independent parts of the world (Cueto 2013; Biehl and Petryna 2013). The precise associations of poverty and disease and disease and development were debated, but technology was frequently considered the solution to disease eradication, which in turn would enable economic development and poverty reduction (McMillen 2015; Cueto 2013). Tackling single diseases was thus often the modus operandi of many public health initiatives, as the histories of malaria, tuberculosis, and smallpox attest—but with smallpox representing the only success story (Greene et al. 2013; Packard 2011; Rhodes 2013). Yet the tail end of the era of international health also saw 134 countries coming together to forge the seminal Alma Ata Declaration of 1978 embracing the tenets of primary health care and promising "health for all by 2000" (Basilico et al. 2013). As Basilico and coauthors argue, however, the election of Thatcher and Reagan soon after, and the consequent inculcation of neoliberalism and its turn toward markets as the basis for economic redistribution and societal problem solving, ensured that Alma Ata would never be implemented and that the role of the private sector would have more prominence in responding to health issues (2013).

Global health thus arose as a facet of neoliberalism and globalization's outcomes including large movements of people, increased income inequality, diminished reach of the state, increasing health and disease disparities between rich and poor nations, and the turn toward privatization in solving social and economic issues (Basilico et al. 2013; Biehl and Petryna 2014). Many of international health's debates remain, including the roles of technology and Western expertise, and for that reason Didier Fassin has called global health more of a "signifier" of change than a distinct break from the era it presumably succeeds (2013, 101). Yet global health does possess a different institutional architecture, with the private sector and highly influential philanthropic organizations such as the Bill and Melinda Gates Foundation (BMGF) joining global organizations like the World Bank and WHO, nongovernmental organizations (NGOs), and state actors in informing which health issues are critical to address and the best way to address them. There are exceptions to the argument that global health overwhelmingly focuses on infectious diseases in low-income countries (Koplan et al. 2009), but there is less debate over the understanding that infectious diseases in the field of global health have again come to constitute critical problems desperately needing intervention, and that such intervention will likely be top-down and Western driven (Biehl and Petryna 2013; 2014). Or, as put in a more historically attuned way by Greene and his colleagues, that "global health priorities in the present have been patterned by social forces with roots in the colonial past" (2013, 34).

Infectious diseases, then, have once again come to the forefront, but not just because of historical influence. The AIDS epidemic reminded a complacent public health constabulary that infectious diseases not only could happen in high- as well as low-income countries, but could prove highly intractable particularly in the face of misguided responses (see Oppenheimer 1988; Kalipeni et al. 1994). AIDS and other infectious diseases have also become security issues, particularly with increased movements of people and the rise of bioterrorism. In the case of tuberculosis, large numbers of individuals arriving in the United States and EU in recent decades from regions where TB is endemic have caused a resurgence of tuberculosis rates and a subsequent turn toward tightened borders and surveillance (Craddock 2008). But it has also galvanized greater awareness of the fact that in many parts of the world, tuberculosis never receded and, in fact, was continuing to devastate lives and economies. The onset of AIDS and its attendant rates of tuberculosis coinfection, as well as the growth of MDR-TB strains worldwide, also gained public health and media attention (Nightingale 2010). The result was the re-creation within Western agencies of tuberculosis as an object of public health urgency that in turn creates a "non-optional duty to act" (Biehl 2011, 106). And yet it is an urgency that never disappeared for those millions living with, or at risk of, the disease.

Recognition that tuberculosis and other infectious disease burdens were part of entrenched poverty and growing global inequality led to the Millennium Summit of world leaders in 2000 and the creation of the Millennium Development Goals (MDGs), a set of eight "time-bound and quantifiable targets for addressing extreme poverty in its many dimensions." Then UN secretary-general Kofi Annan specifically called for member states to work with nonstate actors to tackle extreme poverty and pandemic diseases (Zunz 2012, 284). Goal six of the MDGs was to halt and reverse the incidence of major infectious diseases including tuberculosis by 2015 (Millennium Project 2006). The declaration of these MDGs, in turn, mobilized a set of funding streams and initiatives that could at least in theory begin achieving the ambitions contained in the goals and their targets (Farmer et al. 2013).

Aeras and TB Alliance thus came into being within the context of the MDGs and the reinvigorated initiatives against infectious diseases. They had the direct support of the then director general of the WHO, Gro Brundtland, and the financial backing of the BMGF, the U.S. Agency for International Development (USAID), and EU governments. In embracing technologies as the best way to mitigate, and to eventually vanquish, tuberculosis they work across institutions and agencies, among other things partnering with scientists in academia, industry, and biotech; developing clinical trial sites in high-burden countries to test new drug and vaccine candidates; and negotiating involvement of pharmaceutical industry players. Although I will elaborate on all of these facets of PDP practice in the rest of the book, it is worth answering now the question frequently raised of why the very pharmaceutical industry that has ignored tuberculosis for the past five decades would turn around and help develop TB vaccines and drugs.

The answer is multilayered. First, pharmaceutical practices have placed the industry under more regulatory scrutiny, with negative financial impacts. Increased criticism over industry marketing tactics, inadequate or flawed safety testing, and lack of transparency have resulted in part in tighter control by the Food and Drug Administration (FDA) over new drug approvals (Hughes 2008; Paul et al. 2010). Additionally, most blockbuster drugs are going off patent with no new ones to replace them. With fewer new innovative compounds versus me-too drugs[5] in the development pipeline, generic competition, and significant increases in the cost of producing new drugs,[6] pharmaceutical companies are facing "unprecedented challenges to their business model" (Paul et al. 2010). Pharmaceutical companies have thus been looking for other methods of retaining profit levels, and turning to PDPs for long-term planning has been one way of doing this (and more on that later).

Finally, there is what has come to be called corporate social responsibility (CSR). Contending with negative public opinion by reaching out to communities and doing good is not new to industry. As Bishop and Green (2008) argue, using innovations such as microcredit schemes to tackle social problems, or channeling profits into foundations helping the poor, constitutes a long history of industry participation in aiding society's underclasses. For the pharmaceutical industry, doing good has been going on under different names since at least the 1950s, when the American public, and Congress, became frustrated with rapidly rising prescription drug prices and price fixing (Tobbell 2012). Merck's unlimited donation of its drug mectizan, a treatment for onchocerciasis or river blindness, to any country and anyone who needed it was an early and oft-cited example of pharmaceutical company beneficence to the underserved. Largely unregulated transnational corporate practices in the 1990s, however, were particularly recognized as often exacerbating poverty and harming urban and rural environments in areas of commercial production. One result of this was a public push toward greater recognition on the part of corporations of the impact of their actions, and more effort in implementing initiatives aimed at ameliorating conditions of poverty and environmental degradation (Jenkins 2005). Whatever the motivation, CSR encompasses many different practices from minimal donations to charitable organizations to more meaningful community initiatives or internal restructuring to mitigate detrimental practices (Blowfield and Frynas 2005; Newell 2005). PDPs have become one way for pharmaceutical companies to pursue CSR in various capacities. Some contribute in very superficial ways, while others have actually opened infectious disease research and development departments or units.

These moves into nonlucrative R&D have understandably generated suspicions about pharmaceutical company motivations (see McGoey, Reiss, and Wahlberg 2011). One criticism is that pharmaceutical companies are focusing on infectious diseases as a way to get a foot in the door of new markets in emerging economies such as China and India. After doing so, however, the question becomes whether they will then gradually turn their attention toward those conditions such as hypertension or diabetes more often suffered by middle-class populations in these regions. The short answer to this is yes, they likely will, and they are not hiding this fact. And contrary to the implication, this in itself does not subvert efforts companies put into tuberculosis R&D. Financial motivation behind participation in neglected drug research is not necessarily incommensurate with doing good and moving tuberculosis R&D forward in relevant ways. Pharmaceutical companies are, after all, not charitable organizations. As every drug firm representative indicated to me, they have no intention of going it alone on neglected disease research, because of course ultimately all companies—publicly traded or not—have to consider returns on their investments or else seek external funding for non-lucrative projects, and they have been candid about this position in their negotiations with nonprofit partners. This does put into question the durability of their involvement in tuberculosis efforts, however.

My interviews with those in the pharmaceutical industry were particularly instructive in illustrating the mix of financial motivations, public health need, scientific opportunities, and public relations involved in decisions over neglected disease research. In answer to my question of why a pharmaceutical company would be involved in research on infectious diseases that promise few if any returns on investment, responses typically indicated that it was a mix of CSR as well as an economic objective in eventually tapping into middle-class diseases and markets. As one pharmaceutical executive expounded, however, the hope for profit in the long term was intimately entwined with addressing public health need in the short term. Curing burdens of tuberculosis would in turn reduce government costs and spur economic growth. Meanwhile, pharmaceutical companies would have gained a presence and potentially the ability to expand their business opportunities. In other words, current commitments to improving burdens of infectious disease are not just a ruse for the real goal of access to middle-class constituencies, though this is also important. Instead, each goal serves a separate purpose in negotiating the consumer, shareholder, and business angles of pharmaceutical activity.

The pharmaceutical industry is not monolithic in responding to similar conditions, however. It is composed rather of individual companies that have developed highly variable cultures of ethics and social responsibility and make very different decisions about short- and long-term research goals. As historians of the pharmaceutical industry note, decisions companies make in attempting to rebound during moments of industry crisis are neither obvious nor singular (see Gaudillière 2008; Galambos and Sturchio 1998). Some pharmaceutical companies are choosing not to turn toward infectious disease research, either because they are restructuring in other ways, because they do not have similar social and ethical commitments, or because they choose to act on those commitments through other initiatives. As Sunder Rajan in particular notes in his work on biotechnology (2006), there is not a singular capitalism at work in shaping the coordinates of pharmaceutical and biotechnological production. There are capitalisms in the plural, responding to multivalent and dynamic factors from shifting definitions of the market, scientific imperatives, global financial fluctuations, and public pressures. This in turn, however, makes industry involvement in PDPs more unpredictable and even precarious.

Indeed, several large pharmaceutical companies—namely Novartis, AstraZeneca, and Pfizer—have already exited the tuberculosis research and development endeavor. Novartis has transferred their tuberculosis drug compounds to TB Alliance to "take financial and operational responsibility for continued research" (TB Alliance 2014c), meaning they no longer plan to subsidize or partner with TB Alliance in moving their compounds down the R&D pipeline. All of these companies realized the resources it takes to develop tuberculosis drugs or vaccines and decided they had made the wrong decision in pursuing that line of research regardless of what motivated them in the first place.

One obvious question deriving from motivation is how to think about the contradictions coexisting, however uneasily, within pharmaceutical companies who remain in neglected disease research projects. How do we reconcile these do-good practices with the controversial means these same pharmaceutical companies sometimes employ in developing lucrative pharmaceuticals? The short answer, and the one that pertains to this book, is to recognize that pharmaceutical company efforts as part of PDPs need to be evaluated on their own merits irrespective of the rest of their corporate practices.

Limits and Contestations of PDPs

My focus in this book on the practices, ethics, and innovations constituting humanitarian pharmaceutical production does not obviate the limits to PDPs' potential achievements and the controversies in which they are embedded. One of the biggest factors making tuberculosis PDPs even possible is the influx of philanthropic funding. Philanthropy's association with infectious disease interventions is not new. What is new about the role of philanthropy today is the amount of money foundations have to expend and the degree of influence they wield in making their donations (Bull and McNeill 2007; Zunz 2012). The richest and most visible philanthropic organization operating today is the BMGF. In 2005 the BMGF gave $470 million to support global health initiatives; by 2013 this had grown to $1.3 billion. All other foundations combined gave $600 million the same year (Institute for Health Metrics and Evaluation 2014). As more than one informant has told me, the BMGF more than any other donor has changed the landscape of tuberculosis drug and vaccine research. They essentially created, and overwhelmingly fund, both TB Alliance and Aeras, thus holding responsibility for the number of compounds and vaccines that partnerships have been able to move into the development pipeline.

This very largesse, however, also causes controversy. Criticism has become widespread that BMGF, because of the sheer volume of its donations, has attained inordinate power in shaping what is valorized in global health, and what is not, through its funding decisions. As well as deeming some diseases worthy of intervention and not others, critics point to BMGF's primary focus on technological fixes including drugs, diagnostics, and vaccines, to the detriment of strengthening health-care systems or broader public health interventions (see Farmer et al. 2013). For tuberculosis, a reliance on technologies can seem particularly inadequate given the complex interrelations with social ecologies of deprivation. Yet to this rebuke comes an opposing opinion from Paul Farmer, who in his book *Pathologies of Power* asks the question of "what happens if, after analysis reveals poverty as the root cause of tuberculosis, tuberculosis control strategies ignore the sick and focus solely on eradicating poverty? . . . this ostensibly progressive view would have us ignore both current distress and the tools of modern medicine that might relieve it, thereby committing a new and grave injustice" (2004, 146–47).

To add to this trenchant observation, I elaborate in chapter 2 that the way PDPs approach pharmaceutical development—their attention to upstream and downstream details of community desire, physician attitudes, and logistics of deployment—means that these interventions are not just focused on technological fixes but rather on a much wider field of actors and relations. For PDPs, too, the "grave injustice" mentioned by Farmer already occurred over the last decades of failure on the part of governments, global health organizations, and the pharmaceutical industry to apprehend one of the most devastating diseases ever known. In their minds, they are redressing this injustice.

But another critique of the focus on technology is its embeddedness in the turn toward metrics: focusing on those interventions whose outcomes are readily measured rather than those that might have positive but hard-to-quantify impacts. Like many so-called philanthro-capitalist foundations today whose money comes from corporate earnings, the BMGF approaches its donations along a business model: they want to be able to see returns on their investments. While the results of initiatives with broader social or economic remit are difficult to quantify, new vaccine and drug rollout in high disease-burden communities constitutes some of the most easily measurable improvements in health. This turn to accountability is not unique to BMGF: as Vincanne Adams discusses, many of the major global health institutions including the NIH and the WHO also currently favor those interventions that can be readily proven effective. As she argues, while reliance upon certain metrics of success can make interventions comparable across geographies, they can also leave out the importance of local variation and narrow the definition of what constitutes a successful health intervention (Adams 2013; Merry 2011).

Despite their departure from dominant pharmaceutical development, PDPs also nevertheless are overwhelmingly Western-financed, Western-driven enterprises. As such, questions posed by Jasanoff (2006) and others are valid here of how technologies developed at the initiative of Western countries for the benefit of those in non-Western countries produce new structures of social practice or constitute and reconstitute transnational relations. TB Alliance and Aeras take positive steps to work with local scientists and take the pulse of communities, physicians, and governments of high-burden countries where they intend to distribute successful new therapies. But these actions are not the same thing as asking from the start whether tuberculosis drugs and vaccines are what communities prioritize, how high-burden countries can be brought in as more equal partners, or whether the implementation of new tuberculosis therapies might threaten resource allocations to other health problems.

The critique of Western-centrism and the uneasy power relations inhering in medical interventions especially in postcolonial contexts (Crane 2013) also applies, of course, to humanitarianism. A few words are in order, then, as to how I am using this term. I am in part recognizing that humanitarian practices are themselves political and time-sensitive constructions. The objects of humanitarian attention, while seemingly obvious, actually become visible through the convergence of social, ideological, and historical factors that together shape particular issues into problems (Hacking 1995, cited in Fassin 2012). Right now, as Nikolas Rose (2006) among many have noted, recent advances in genetic research in particular has meant a political turn—or return—to the biological with its promise and potential for ameliorating life. This turn also characterizes humanitarianism, where for instance the NGO MSF has been successful in evidencing the burdens of disease among disenfranchised populations and the suffering it adds to already precarious lives (see Redfield 2013). Similarly, individuals living with tuberculosis have gained traction through their disease and its attendant suffering, where their status as poor did little to garner assistance. Precarious lives thus materialize out of this precise moral and political valence. As Fassin astutely notes, "tensions between the relation of inequality and solidarity, and between a relation of domination and a relation of assistance, is constitutive of all humanitarian government" (2012, 3).

Pharmaceutical humanitarianism is somewhat different in that it does not focus on a particular population or region. Through the dissemination of technologies, pharmaceutical humanitarianism applies a broad-based antidote to widespread suffering. The primary tension I am concerned with here is not the object of pharmaceutical humanitarianism, that is, producing new and better therapies for tuberculosis. It is in how that endeavor might play out for the intended recipients and their governments and caregivers, and how predetermined those relations are in the very structure of PDP governance. Whether and how much communities and local governments will have a strong say in how they apprehend the new technologies—how the implementation process will take into account that the poor do not just experience adversity but also respond to it in definitive ways (Chandhoke 2012)—remains to be seen. There is also a question of the time-sensitivity of philanthropic and humanitarian aid: How long will tuberculosis be deemed worthy of intervention? And when that time is done—when factors converge to create other issues as urgent problems—then what will become of PDPs and the disease they are striving so hard to defeat? The answer to this question is found in part in the following chapters.

The research I did for this book involved six years of multisited ethnography. A large part of the information I gathered came from the eighty or so in-depth interviews I conducted with TB Alliance and Aeras CEOs, medical, communication, and sales officers, and scientists; directors of pharmaceutical departments focused on neglected disease research; pharmaceutical company scientists; WHO officials; BMGF and MSF representatives; biotech and university scientists; and other nonprofit and NGO representatives partnered with TB Alliance and Aeras or involved in tuberculosis research and development. Other important sources of information were the conferences I attended, particularly the five annual Union World Conferences on Lung Health held between 2010 and 2014, the Global Vaccine Forum, and an International Vaccine Forum. These gave me the opportunity to attend sessions to hear the latest in drug and vaccine development, but also provided key insights from audience questions as well as discussions. I also informally interviewed researchers, public health officials, and clinicians attending these conferences from all over the world. From these individuals I got a better sense of how particular technologies or organizations worked in their own local settings, and how overarching policies of organizations such as the WHO or BMGF changed in the context of underfunded health systems, inadequate health-care personnel, and variable structures of government command and responsibility.

In 2012 I visited a tuberculosis vaccine clinical trial site outside of Cape Town, South Africa, run by the South African Tuberculosis Vaccine Initiative (SATVI). I toured their facilities and interviewed researchers, staff, a community advisory board facilitator, clinic administrator, and hospital administrator. I toured three pharmaceutical production facilities: the GSK vaccine facility outside of Brussels, Belgium; the GSK Drugs for the Developing World (DDW) facility outside of Madrid, Spain; and Aeras's headquarters and vaccine manufacturing facility outside of Washington, D.C. During each of these visits I received extensive tours of the various labs, production facilities, quality assurance rooms, and in the case of the DDW, the automated screening "factory" in the chemical library. I also interviewed numerous scientists working at each of these facilities about what was being researched and developed, how, and with what other partners or funding sources.

Finally, I also scanned PDP and pharmaceutical websites with regularity, reading how each organization or company described what they do and the mission they embrace, but also reading annual reports, news releases, and linked scientific publications. I subscribed to pharmacology and access-to-medicines listservs and conducted secondary literature reviews.

Virtually everyone with whom I interacted—through my interviews, tours, conversations, etc.—was more than happy to provide me with the information I was seeking. It became clear early on that everyone was not only dedicated to what they were doing and trying to achieve, but that they wanted others to know about their efforts, too. I had to remind people often that I was a social scientist: I was there to put relations and practices into broader contexts, not necessarily to advocate. I don't think I could have undertaken the research for this book, however, without fundamentally believing in what these PDPs and their partners were trying to achieve. And there were a few times when I was not able to get information I wanted. Just because PDPs are noncommercial does not mean they are nonproprietary. If I asked too much about a candidate drug or vaccine that they weren't ready to make public, the conversation was shut down. This did not happen often, but it reminded me that I was still researching arenas that were not entirely open to everyone. PDPs do not function along the approach that everything they produce will be part of the commons; they control what they produce, but in a particular way— that is, to ensure their products remain affordable.

I utilize all of this information in the following chapters to examine how partnerships are formed and maintained, the IP configurations assumed, and the precariousness of financing; the innovations in science when profit incentives are not constraining time and research trajectories, reconfigurations of failure, the scope of success, and collaborations across industries and disciplines; and the difference PDPs make to clinical trial designs, the new set of ethical questions they bring to the table, the impacts of trials beyond participants and trial communities, the constraints of regulatory requirements, and limits to innovative clinical trial design.

I draw inspiration for my analysis from James Ferguson's article "The Uses of Neoliberalism" (2010) where he recommends that critical scholars pause in enumerating the pitfalls of neoliberal capitalism and ask instead what benefits some initiatives are having even if they are not changing paradigms. PDPs do not exist explicitly to change the paradigm of pharmaceutical production in twenty-first-century capitalism, yet they are doing so in their own right by redirecting logics of production through the altered stakes and apparatuses of humanitarian conduct. Their efforts indirectly bring visibility to what is deeply wrong about current pharmaceutical economies, while more directly providing a way forward—for the industry itself, and for the millions with tuberculosis.

1 THE POSSIBILITIES AND PARAMETERS
OF DRUG AND VACCINE PARTNERSHIPS

IN FEBRUARY 2000, a group of 120 concerned scientists, academics, non-profit agencies, industry representatives, government representatives, and donors met in Cape Town, South Africa, to discuss the problem of tuberculosis and its possible solutions. The formal outcome of that meeting coalesced in October of that year in Bangkok, when the not-for-profit TB Alliance was announced by Dr. Gro Harlem Brundtland, the then director of the WHO (www.tballiance.org). TB Alliance is the primary organization focused on developing affordable antituberculosis drugs. It is something of a "virtual" organization—the term used by its former chief medical officer, Ann Ginsberg—contracting with academic and private sector researchers rather than building their own laboratories, and seeking collaborations with both biotech and pharmaceutical partners in pursuing improved treatments for drug-susceptible and drug-resistant tuberculosis, including those coinfected with TB and HIV.

The primary organization spearheading tuberculosis vaccine development is Aeras. Aeras had its beginnings in the small biotechnology firm Sequella, which focused its attention on TB drugs and anti-infectives until the BMGF approached them with an interest in vaccines for TB. The Sequella Foundation formed in 1999 in response to this interest, and a relationship was forged with the University of Cape Town to assist with development of vaccines and with clinical trials of successful candidates. By 2003, the Sequella Foundation wanted to create a separate entity for this endeavor, and Aeras emerged (Peg Willingham, former senior director of external affairs, Aeras, personal communication, June 16, 2010). Aeras is more "bricks and mortar" (Ginsberg, personal communication, December 6, 2011) than TB Alliance in the way it operates, with sleek headquarters outside of Washington, D.C., incorporating its own labs, biostatistics group, clinical monitors, and manufacturing facility.[1] That has some implications in what they look for in partners given how much they do internally. Yet philosophically Aeras is very similar to TB Alliance in "looking around the world for expertise they need, facilities or trial sites or populations they need to get their products from the lab bench to the patients at the end" with a "common line drawn in the sand that any partner has to agree that any product will be made affordable" to populations in low-income countries (Ginsberg, personal communication, December 6, 2011).

My intention in this chapter is not to exhaustively describe all current partnerships in TB drug or vaccine production, but rather to highlight those collaborations illustrating the key players and relations constituting PDP research and development. My primary argument in this chapter is that the particular contingencies of humanitarian pharmaceutical production demand a fluidity in the partnerships PDPs form, a constant negotiation of who will join or exit the development process and what role each partner will play. There is an excitement in the field of tuberculosis research now, galvanized by donor funding and the first set of vaccine candidates and drug compounds to come down the R&D pipeline in decades. Yet this enthusiasm is matched by concern regarding the slow speed of developments, precarious funding, and the skittish involvement of industry. As to this last factor, the necessity in the PDP model of bringing together highly disparate players with distinct motivations for working toward tuberculosis vaccine and drug development ultimately raises the question of what "partnership" means and for whom. The very term, like that of "collaboration," suggests compatibility and cohesion, and as such often masks the degree to which inequalities of power characterize collaborations (Crane 2014) including those forged by PDPs. It also suggests a certain solidity of purpose, indicating nothing about the sometimes tenuous circumstances under which relationships are held together.

Power relations and diverse motivations do not translate necessarily into diminished outcomes. As Anna Tsing describes in her book *Friction: An Ethnography of Global Connection* (2004), actors who typically maintain competing if not conflicting agendas can come together, and the friction they produce in negotiating common goals from different positions and motivations can be highly productive—"the stuff of emergent politics" as they create the political, scientific, or financial conditions to move beyond entrenched ways of seeing and responding (2004, 247). Tuberculosis PDPs hold this potential for "productive friction" as they negotiate new modes of production and scientific-experimental practices that make them sites of economic and biomedical innovation beyond their success in generating new interventions. The friction remains productive as long as the divergent agendas brought to the table remain in alignment toward the common goal of new vaccine and drug production. Yet Tsing also recognizes that collaborations hold within their very infrastructure the threat of cooptation as funders or international organizations wield their inequitable degrees of power and when ideas—in this case, of intervention or R&D processes—get "imagined and imposed" by particular actors to the exclusion of others or to the collective (2004, 264). Friction becomes less productive as well when motivations produce contradictory rather than compatible end goals.

Flexible Productions

In TB Alliance's early days, the fact that tuberculosis is caused by a bacterium played to the organization's advantage for two reasons. The first of these is that antibiotics already on the market and prescribed for other bacterial infections hold the possibility for efficacy in treating tuberculosis.[2] The first approach TB Alliance took upon its inception, then, was to search for "low hanging fruit" as TB Alliance's former manager of communications, Derek Ambrosino, put it (personal communication, February 23, 2009)—that is, approaching pharmaceutical companies for permission to take existing antibiotics and test their applicability toward tuberculosis. One example of this approach is moxifloxacin, an antibiotic owned by Bayer Pharmaceuticals of Germany and already on the market to treat acute respiratory infections. Since the drug is already patented and FDA-approved, TB Alliance moved past some of the early and time-consuming studies to establish safety data and went directly to a Phase III clinical trial named REMox (www.tballiance.org).

REMox was designed to ascertain whether substituting moxifloxacin for either isoniazid or rifampicin—both part of first-line drug regimens—would shorten treatment time from six to four months. If successful, it would have resulted in what TB Alliance touted as "registration of the first new drug approved for the treatment of drug-sensitive TB in nearly fifty years" (www.tballiance.org). Bayer agreed to supply the drug free of charge for the trial, a relatively small price to pay since they would have retained all rights to moxifloxacin after the trial and gained another use for it if the drug proved successful. This, even though TB Alliance paid for the trial enabling the expanded market for the relatively short time remaining on moxifloxacin's patent (Elizabeth Gardiner, former vice president of market access, TB Alliance, personal communication, October 29, 2012). However, the trial proved unsuccessful in reaching its objective of a four-month drug treatment time.[3]

A similar low-hanging fruit, or drug repurposing, scheme is happening at GSK's DDW facility in Tres Cantos, Spain, which has a relationship with TB Alliance in some of its research and development. There, researchers are going back to a large class of antibiotics, beta-lactams or b-lactams, to investigate their efficacy against *M. tuberculosis*. B-lactams are broad-spectrum antibiotics, meaning they are effective against a wide range of bacteria. Dr. David Barros-Aguirre of GSK and colleagues are performing a number of laboratory experiments that so far are showing the ability of beta-lactams to kill mycobacteria very quickly. One in particular, meropenem, was administered in early-stage human trials in South Africa with very optimistic results (Diacon et al. 2016). This success in turn has garnered new funding from the BMGF to look at other b-lactams for their success against *M. tuberculosis* (Barros-Aguirre, personal communication, June 27, 2014 and July 18, 2016).

In more recent years, TB Alliance has shifted away from a focus on low-hanging fruits to an emphasis on fostering new compound discovery and development, and pharmaceutical companies in turn have played varied but proactive roles in these endeavors. Mary Moran (2005) argues in her study of public–private partnerships in neglected disease drug development that many pharmaceutical companies have changed the nature of their involvement in collaborations from an emphasis on late-stage product in the early years to one emphasizing upstream compound development. Part of the reason for this switch, according to Moran, is that upstream research is less expensive and therefore better tolerated by shareholders nervous about supporting initiatives with low potential for return on investments. It is in the later and more expensive stages of compound development that partners such as TB Alliance play key roles as they apply their resources toward moving compounds further down the pipeline.

Yet in the early 2000s some pharmaceutical companies such as Novartis, GSK, Eli Lilly, AstraZeneca, and Sanofi made decisions to open research centers or to support company offshoots or departments specifically devoted to developing new infectious disease drugs and vaccines from the preclinical to the manufacturing and marketing stage. Which diseases these new initiatives pursue, or pursued, is often determined by what was already in the company portfolio or by the compounds acquired through acquisition of other companies. Why potentially effective compounds against unprofitable infectious diseases exist in the first place in industry pipelines varies. Sometimes they were part of smaller biotech companies' development of niche areas of expertise or because models indicated adequate markets for their development. Other times, researchers using older scientific methods of drug discovery entailing a degree of trial and error in screening molecular compounds against disease discovered promising tuberculosis drug or vaccine candidates by accident in the process of searching for compounds effective against other conditions such as cancer.

Either way, these compounds are now helping buttress the new initiatives of the last decade or so. Yet very few pharmaceutical companies are willing to go it alone in financing tuberculosis drug compounds or vaccines all the way to market. Japan's Otsuka Pharmaceuticals is the only exception to this, having developed their one tuberculosis drug, delamanid, all the way up to its current status in Phase III trials. More will be said about this in the following two chapters. For the remaining pharmaceutical companies, forging collaborations with TB Alliance enables them to gain assistance in the design and financing of late-stage clinical trials as well as regulatory expertise with promising drug candidates. The compound bedaquiline and its developer, Janssen, represent an example of this way forward. I go into some detail on this particular partnership because it evidences the precariousness of PDP collaborations, but also the dexterity of PDP operational capacities and the ability to turn precariousness into productivity. Describing bedaquiline's pathway also highlights some of the challenges of *M. tuberculosis*: the deficit of knowledge about the bacterium over the many years of neglect now means that much is not known about how the bacterium acts inside the body or which immune responses are effective against it.

Bedaquiline is a promising drug with a new mechanism of action against tuberculosis—that is, a way of interfering with *M. tuberculosis* that is different from existing drugs. Like HIV, *M. tuberculosis* is a fast-mutating pathogen, and intervening effectively in it requires not just more than one drug but a drug regimen that targets different aspects of the bacterium. Presently there are six categories of antituberculosis compounds in clinical trials, namely fluoroquinolones, nitroimidazoles, diarylquinolines, rifamycins, oxazolidinones, and ethylenediamines, and all of these work differently at the cellular level (Ma et al. 2010). Bedaquiline belongs to the diarylquinoline category, and its new mechanism of action involves inhibiting ATP-synthase3, a factor in *M. tuberculosis*'s energy production. As articulated by David McNeely, the former medical leader in charge of developing bedaquiline, the drug is "starving the bacterium" and thus critically intervening in its ability to reproduce (personal communication, August 14, 2009).

Janssen is an offshoot of the pharmaceutical company Johnson & Johnson, dedicated to developing novel treatments for infectious diseases such as HIV, Hepatitis C, and tuberculosis. Like most industry offshoots focused on infectious disease drug and vaccine development, Janssen is connected to its parent company but by definition of its mission operates under different rules for making research and development decisions. Most of these offshoot initiatives are not expected to turn profits like their parent companies, but this means depending on a mixture of subsidization, collaboration, and diversified research pipelines to drive their innovations. Janssen, for example, includes ARVs in its research portfolio. ARVs constitute "crossover" drugs sustaining sizeable profits in high-income markets even though the majority of HIV-positive individuals live in low-income regions. Profits from ARVs can then subsidize research into less profitable diseases like tuberculosis. Johnson & Johnson, "recognizing the public health value" of tuberculosis drugs, also channels money to Janssen for their tuberculosis and other drug development, but Janssen nevertheless formed a partnership with TB Alliance in order to offset clinical trial costs and to expand adoption potential of bedaquiline.

Contrary to the perception that major pharmaceutical companies only recently turned their attention to infectious diseases, Janssen has already invested a significant amount of time and resources in developing bedaquiline. Before collaborating with TB Alliance, they advanced the compound through smaller Phase I and Phase II safety trials before determining that it was ready to be tested in larger Phase IIb trials to ascertain correct dosing as well as efficacy. One highly desirable property of bedaquiline is that it works on both latent as well as actively replicating forms of the bacilli—a relatively unique property since most tuberculosis treatments act on one form or another but not both (McNeely, personal communication, August 14, 2009). Dormant bacteria, though also found in cases of active TB, characterize those with latent tuberculosis, where bacteria are not actively replicating or being transmitted to other individuals but nevertheless remain viable in the lungs of their host and are able to become active if the immune system is compromised. Given that an estimated two billion people live with latent tuberculosis, of which 5 to 10 percent will develop active TB over the course of a lifetime, a better understanding of the metabolic and physiological strategies used by bacteria in the dormant phase is a critical component to designing sterilizing drugs, that is, drugs that can target dormant bacteria. This is made even more critical because dormant cells are responsible for relapse, so the "whole challenge is to kill them so that when people are cured, they are really cured," as the senior science advisor of the WHO Stop TB Partnership, Christian Lienhardt, put it to me (personal communication, December 9, 2010). Janssen's partnership with TB Alliance enabled it to conduct late-stage—that is, Phase IIb—clinical trials of efficacy against drug-resistant and drug-sensitive strains of *M. tuberculosis* (Ambrosino, personal communication, July 29, 2009).

In this instance, TB Alliance and Janssen divided rights to bedaquiline not along tuberculosis versus other antibacterial applications, but rather along lines of drug-susceptible and MDR-TB. Perhaps surprisingly, Janssen assumed rights over bedaquiline for the smaller MDR-TB market. In this case, it was not the size of the market that mattered as much as the expense of clinical trials and the time to market. When effective therapies already exist, as they do in tuberculosis, new drugs need to prove that they are at least as effective as currently existing regimens or that they present another advantage over existing therapies if they want FDA approval. Late-stage clinical trials for drug-susceptible tuberculosis thus need to enroll higher numbers of participants in order to statistically prove that a new drug is at least as effective as the current four-drug regimen.

For tuberculosis, proving that a new drug contributes to shortening treatment from six to four months requires tracking participants for at least two years to record relapse rates. This is because tuberculosis has no known biomarker.[4] Typically in trials of vaccine (or drug) candidates for other infectious diseases, you have a biomarker—that is, a measurable change in the body that signals, or correlates with, the immunological reaction known to confer protection against the disease in question. An example of this would be measuring CD4 counts or viral loads in HIV-positive individuals during trials of ARV drug efficacy: if viral loads go down or CD4 counts go up among those individuals receiving the new drug, these are signs that the drug is working. It makes clinical trials simpler to run and facilitates speedier accumulation of necessary data. Not having a biomarker for tuberculosis complicates research and makes clinical trials lengthier, because of the long follow up, and thus more expensive (Uli Fruth, secretary of the Vaccines Working Group, WHO, personal communication, October 20, 2010).

Proving superiority of a new drug as part of a treatment regimen in MDR-TB is thus much easier given the lower efficacy rates of second-line tuberculosis drugs. Janssen accordingly conducted Phase IIb trials among MDR-TB patients across sites in Thailand, Latvia, Peru, South Africa, and Brazil—all areas with high MDR-TB burdens (McNeely, personal communication, August 14, 2009). Those trials ended by 2012, with results positive enough for Janssen to seek, and receive, early regulatory approval from the FDA and subsequently from Europe's counterpart, the European Medicines Agency (EMA). The FDA awarded Janssen the early approval by the end of 2012, with the caveat that it could only be used in populations of MDR-TB patients who had no other options and that Janssen had to begin Phase III trials within a year in order to further test the drug in larger numbers of trial participants and to address unanswered questions about why there was a slightly higher mortality rate among participants receiving bedaquiline in the Phase IIb trial versus those receiving a standard regimen for MDR-TB (Lessem 2014a). In this instance, TB Alliance did not provide Janssen direct subsidization for drug development. Janssen financed its own Phase IIb trial but relied upon TB Alliance to work with the WHO as well as various regional regulatory agencies and national health ministries to pave the way for bedaquiline to be adopted by assisting in the registration process and helping national tuberculosis programs with implementation plans. As McNeely noted, pharmaceutical companies "don't do this health policy" kind of work—it is not part of a commercial approach. As he summarized it, the compound itself, rather than Janssen, is what gains from a relationship with TB Alliance (McNeely, personal communication, August 14, 2009).

This relationship, however, also illustrates the tenuous hold TB Alliance has over its collaborators and, like its arrangement with Bayer, begs the question of what "partnership" actually means in the context of highly discrepant interests and institutional practices. To work with any partner, including a pharmaceutical company, TB Alliance requires them to commit to their "AAA strategy" of affordability, access, and availability should drugs prove efficacious enough for adoption. Janssen was no exception, and its own initiative in pursuing tuberculosis research and development lent them a degree of trustworthiness. As articulated in 2011 by Elizabeth Gardiner, former vice president of market access for TB Alliance, it was "remarkable that Janssen is out there producing a tuberculosis drug" given the lack of economic incentive. Citing a recent MSF report naming MDR-TB as one example where it makes sense to have a single drug supplier because of limited market—something that typically drives up the price of a pharmaceutical given the lack of competition—Gardiner concurred that few in the TB drug development community are worried about a company like Janssen having marketing control over a new drug for MDR-TB (Gardiner, personal communication, November 29, 2011).

Yet this optimism proved unfounded. Once bedaquiline—brand name Sirturo—received FDA approval in late 2012, Janssen priced the drug well beyond the capabilities of most individuals to purchase it: a course of bedaquiline costs $900 in low-income countries and $26,000 in high-income countries. Its price tag even jeopardizes the ability of countries to purchase the drug in bulk for its populations with MDR-TB, or for procurement agencies such as the WHO's Global Drug Facility to distribute it effectively given lack of demand (Lessem 2014a). It is puzzling why Janssen would bother to develop a drug with an overwhelmingly poor consumer base and then price it for a high-income market, virtually ensuring a lack of sales. But it also made clear the fact that ultimately, TB Alliance had no control over what Janssen, and by extension, Johnson & Johnson, did with a drug they developed themselves.

But that is not the end of the story. TB Alliance is adroitly capitalizing on two facets of proprietary rulings that essentially allow them to sidestep Janssen's intransigence: the first is to seek approval for a drug regimen rather than a single drug; and the second—which follows from the first—is to seek approval for a different indication. TB Alliance, then, tested bedaquiline (B) as part of a drug regimen, BPaZ, along with two other drugs: pyrazinamide (Z), a first-line drug; and one of its own drug compounds, PA-824, now called pretomanid (Pa). They first moved these three compounds into two-week Phase IIa clinical trials in Cape Town, South Africa, enrolling drug-susceptible individuals with high *M. tuberculosis* bacterial counts and testing whether bacterial loads decreased over the course of two weeks. The trial showed that these three drugs in combination killed more than 99 percent of bacteria within this fourteen-day time frame (Andreas Diacon, Stellenbosch University and CEO, TASK Applied Science, personal communication, March 25, 2011).

Now TB Alliance is conducting Phase IIb trials of this regimen in

Tanzania, South Africa, and Uganda to test its efficacy among individuals with drug-susceptible tuberculosis, but also among individuals with some forms of MDR-TB (www.tballiance.org). TB Alliance is able to include MDR-TB patients in its latest clinical trials precisely because they are seeking approval from the FDA for these three drugs as a regimen, not as a combination of three drugs. More will be said about the novelty and importance of drug regimen approval in the next chapter, but the point to make here is that once approved, regimens become distinct products: they are no longer a combination of three particular drugs, but rather an entity that is efficacious only because of molecular interactions happening in tandem. Such a drug regimen as BPaZ, with two new compounds each with different mechanisms of action, furthermore makes almost irrelevant the distinction between drug-susceptible and drug-resistant tuberculosis.[5] It starts with an almost clean slate, so to speak, because MDR-TB is defined as resistance to two of the frontline drugs, isoniazid or rifampicin, neither of which BPaZ contains. With a regimen and an indication for tuberculosis as a whole rather than for MDR-TB, TB Alliance thus reclaims a chance to utilize bedaquiline in a productive way in line with their AAA mission (Ambrosino, personal communication, October 7, 2014).

Though this example would seem to suggest something less than a partnership, much less a productive collaboration, it might be seen another way. Janssen did share its compound with TB Alliance before it was approved. That suggests a level of trust and a willingness to share scientific discovery in a way incommensurate with mainstream pharmaceutical practices, even if neither side ended up holding to the terms of the original arrangement. It was a productive coming together for TB Alliance because they inherited a drug compound that was already well along the pipeline and had shown promising test results. It illustrates well Tsing's argument that friction—in this case, between two agencies with highly divergent ultimate agendas in drug development—can nevertheless be productive even if the collaboratory moment is of brief duration.

Bedaquiline's divergent pathway between TB Alliance and Janssen also highlights the different relations that characterize humanitarian pharmaceutical production. Within that, it illustrates the critical distinction in how both TB Alliance and Aeras handle proprietary claims. Janssen, as part of a commercial company though ostensibly different from it in tackling infectious diseases, proceeded along the standard route predictable for mainstream drug development: they took the fastest and easiest path to approval by focusing on MDR-TB patients, and once they received approval, they marketed bedaquiline basically as Johnson & Johnson would market any of its drugs. Standard regulatory, experimental, and marketing procedures applied, in other words. The faster the time to approval and to market, the greater potential for making profit given that the twenty-year time limit begins at the time the patent is awarded, not when a drug is first marketed. With TB Alliance the end goal was not time-to-market. The value that drives their compound development is how many bodies they can reach with new therapies, and this in turn determines the variant research, regulatory, and proprietary pathways and the very different product they will ultimately derive. Not the shortest path to approval, in other words, but the one maximizing the numbers reached; innovative regulatory policies that shave time off of approval in the interests of saving more lives, as well as money; and, if successful, a patent on a drug regimen that will be used to ensure low rather than high prices, and to preclude other companies—including Johnson & Johnson—from usurping its political-humanitarian purpose. Unlike some alternative commodity development initiatives that utilize the commons to pool new discoveries and keep them open for all to use, TB Alliance and Aeras are proprietary organizations using patents to maintain control over their products. In the case of bedaquiline a patent was desirable to ensure maximum utility in the face of intransigent corporate partners.

But in addition to their relationships with Western pharmaceutical and biotech companies, a strategic facet of TB Alliance's ability to expand the reach of their research and development and to leverage limited resources is the ties they are cultivating with major emerging economies, especially China. An example is their Memorandum of Understanding signed in 2011 with the International Scientific Exchange Foundation of China (ISEFC) to help develop the Global Health Research and Development Center of China (GHRC). GHRC will be the first PDP in China dedicated to "developing new tools that will help address neglected diseases and improve health in China and around the world" (TB Alliance 2011). Targeting BRICS countries is an important strategy for TB Alliance given that Brazil, Russia, India, China, and South Africa all have high burdens of tuberculosis combined with sufficient resources to develop the capacity for drug production for both domestic and regional consumption.

Yet as indicated to me by Mel Spigelman, CEO of TB Alliance, all BRICS countries are very different in what governments want and in the mix of private and public health-care systems or pharmaceutical industries. In other words, as he succinctly summarized it, "all good partnerships are local." For China, then, TB Alliance knew that there would be an expectation on the part of the government to have a majority stake in any collaboration, that—as Spigelman put it—"you couldn't just parachute in" and impose alternative models for drug production. So TB Alliance focused on the ISEFC as a Chinese-owned, not-for-profit entity and attracted local seed funding and worked with the ISEFC to establish the GHRC as China's first PDP. The next stage will be hiring personnel and organizing an independent board with TB Alliance as one partner but with significant buy-in from all constituencies from the Chinese government to the private wealthy sectors (Spigelman, personal communication, December 7, 2011). The initial push will be providing the Chinese population with new tuberculosis drug regimens, with eventual export to neighboring high-burden countries constituting the subsequent goal. TB Alliance is also in conversation with health-care officials in Brazil and India, but agreements have so far not been completed.

TB Alliance joins many corporations, then, in turning to BRICS countries and China in particular for ways to expand their R&D and manufacturing capacities and their markets. Yet unlike most corporations, TB Alliance is not looking for inexpensive labor, lax regulatory and environmental policies, and other investment incentives. China—and ultimately other BRICS countries—hold a potentially pivotal role in the future of PDPs who are currently dependent on donations, however generous. As mentioned in the introduction, the object of philanthropic and humanitarian largesse is shaped through particular political, social, and historical convergences, and they are therefore time sensitive. Donations also only go so far. What China offers is a particularly promising interrelation of science, expertise, infrastructure, industrial capacity, and government support to allow TB Alliance to expand its own capabilities well beyond what has heretofore been possible. With the Chinese government sponsoring the process, tuberculosis drugs can be developed, tested, and manufactured at the scale necessary for China's huge number of patients with tuberculosis, and eventually for export to high-burden countries in Southeast Asia. In making clear the terms of collaboration and, specifically, the role Chinese governmental and nongovernmental agencies will play, China is also all but assuring a more equitable geopolitical balance in its relationship with TB Alliance and the technologies they coproduce.

Clearly, this collaboration bears little resemblance to the one with Janssen. Yet the parallel comes from seeing that the collaboration with

China, like Janssen, turned normative relations of development and production on their head. China, like other BRICS countries, possesses a growing middle class, established education systems, manufacturing sectors, and a large underclass that together are ideal for corporations to expand their markets, manufacturing capacities, and profits. TB Alliance instead is turning to China's government and its resources as a way to expand their ability to reach and assist the underclasses through government-subsidized and government-distributed tuberculosis drugs. The particular set of relations is different in this case than the ones constituting the partnership with Janssen, but they are both mobilizing a similar outcome.

Reworking Vaccine Ecosystems

In the course of my conversation with Joris Vandeputte, senior vice president for Advocacy and Resource Mobilisation for the Dutch-based Tuberculosis Vaccine Initiative (TBVI), he reminded me that collaborative efforts within the vaccine industry are not new. In contrast to the drug industry, he suggested, the vaccine industry "has been doing low-cost development for fifty years" with researchers, producers, and global agencies like the United Nations Children's Fund (UNICEF) working together to get vaccines for infectious diseases from smallpox to influenza developed and disseminated as widely as possible (personal communication, December 8, 2010). This sentiment was echoed by Jim Connolly, former CEO of Aeras, and also formerly the executive vice president of vaccines at Wyeth. As he put it, at the end of the day the mission at Wyeth was not so different than at Aeras—it was to make vaccines (in Wyeth's case, the pneumococcal vaccine) as widely available as possible using whatever financial mechanisms and collaborative arrangements worked to make this happen. Vaccine networks, he continued, are good examples of organizations, including major pharmaceutical companies, willing to come up with low-cost, high-yield products even when it means very low profit margins (Connolly, personal communication, November 18, 2011).

Collaboration in vaccine production in terms of disease targets nonetheless has had its limits outside of the PDP model. Industry has understandably focused their energies predominantly on indications with broad dissemination across low- and high-income markets, such as influenza, HPV, or pneumococcal vaccines. Only within the last decade or so has attention turned once again to a new and better vaccine for tuberculosis with the advent of PDPs. As many researchers in the field point out, however, the last ten years have been remarkable for the number of vaccine candidates already making their way down the research and development pipeline—a total currently of sixteen (Frick 2014). Tuberculosis vaccine PDPs are not just about producing vaccine candidates where recently there were none, critical though that endeavor is to their existence. They are also, like their drug counterparts, attentive to the broader relations—or vaccine ecosystem, as one member of Aeras calls it—that includes regulatory, distribution, financing, and implementation facets posing challenges at least as daunting as the research and development processes. Aeras and its partners, in addressing these challenges, are in significant ways revising longer-standing collaborative models of vaccine production.

The first tuberculosis vaccine to go into efficacy trials since 1968, MVA85A was the particular brainchild of Professor Helen McShane of the Jenner Institute, Oxford University. Evidencing the productive scientific exchanges across different disease fields, McShane noticed that the work on malaria of her PhD supervisor, Professor Adrian Hill, and specifically his work on immune responses in mice, would be pertinent for tuberculosis. McShane translated the relevant immune responses into a tuberculosis vaccine using a viral vector. MVA in the MVA85A vaccine stands for Modified Vaccinia Ankara, a highly attenuated strain of vaccinia (smallpox) virus that has proven an effective vector for delivering proteins to the immune system; 85A is one among many proteins on the surface of *M. tuberculosis*. Proteins, in turn, are the substances, or antigens, that stimulate the immune system to respond to intrusive pathogens such as bacteria.

As McShane explains, in tuberculosis, even if the specifics of effective immune responses are not yet known, it is clear that T cells play an important role in combating the bacterium. So making an effective booster vaccine must entail taking proteins from the current BCG vaccine—made from weakened *Mycobacterium bovis*—or from *M. tuberculosis*, which then stimulate T cells in the body via the virus vector. As stated by Dr. Steve Lockhart, formerly of Emergent BioSolutions, it is a "slightly magic thing," that if you give an antigen or challenge to a person more than once, you often get immune responses that are boosted. But if you give an antigen the second time using a different delivery method—in this case the viral vector following BCG—then you frequently see even better boosting than if you use the same delivery system twice (personal communication, February 16, 2012).

In 2001 McShane received funding from the Wellcome Trust to move MVA85A into early clinical trials. Wellcome, along with BMGF, was one of the first entities funding tuberculosis research, and up until that point there had been little progress in tuberculosis vaccines beyond the mouse stage (McShane, personal communication, July 9, 2012). Testing tuberculosis vaccines in humans is especially difficult: first because good animal models do not exist and therefore animal studies are not particularly predictive in tuberculosis; and second because of the Koch response, an immune reaction that induces immunopathology—inflammation that is detrimental rather than positive. Those with latent TB or who have received the BCG vaccine are especially vulnerable to this response (McShane, personal communication, July 9, 2012). So Phase I and II trials of MVA85A to test its safety (not efficacy) proceeded with huge caution, first being tested in those who did not have the BCG vaccine in the UK, then those who did, and from there moving through successively more targeted populations of HIV-infected, TB-infected, and coinfected adults, then adolescents, and finally infants.

Early-stage clinical trials can be challenging given strict recruitment criteria and the large number of trials needed—in the case of tuberculosis, across geographic, age, coinfection, and vaccination constituencies—to satisfy regulatory and internal requirements for safety. The small number of participants, however, means that academic budgets or grants can cover their expenses when vaccine candidates emerge from academic labs; or in the case of industry, it means they are generally willing to expend the resources on their internal vaccine candidates. Beyond early-stage trials, however, this changes, but not just because more money is needed. Part of the logistics of partnerships in late-stage trials is finding a manufacturer capable of scaling up production of the vaccine—not just for the purposes of later-stage clinical trials, but in the event that the vaccine proves successful. For a tuberculosis vaccine, this means donors are hesitant to fund a late-stage trial until the ability to manufacture a vaccine candidate in excess of one hundred million doses a year is proven (Lockhart, personal communication, February 16, 2012).

Oxford thus turned to Emergent BioSolutions, a small biotech company specializing in vaccines, to address that question, and the Oxford-Emergent Tuberculosis Consortium was forged. The consortium, in turn, signed an agreement with the German biopharmaceutical company

Probiogen in 2009 to license their cell line derived from duck embryonic retinal cells, to enable scaling up of MVA85A manufacturing that until that point had been done laboriously and expensively in small batches using chick embryos (Emergent BioSolutions 2009; Lockhart, personal communication, February 16, 2012). To help pay for and conduct larger Phase IIb clinical trials, Aeras and Wellcome joined as participants in the collaboration, and in July 2009 the trial began in Worcester, outside of Cape Town, South Africa. Run by the SATVI, it enrolled around 2,800 infants, half of whom received the BCG vaccine with a subsequent placebo booster shot, while the other half received BCG and MVA85A as a booster. Unfortunately, by 2013 it was announced that MVA85A failed to show ability to confer heightened protection.

An example of a very different collaborative vaccine production is M72, a vaccine that GSK began developing in the early 2000s. As explained by Gérald Voss, director of the vaccine unit outside of Brussels, M72 is a recombinant vaccine designed to prevent new infections as well as prevent reactivated disease from latent infection, which so far in early clinical trials has shown significant stimulation of CD4 T cells (personal communication, July 6, 2012; Graves and Hokey 2011). GSK is one of only a few pharmaceutical companies researching and developing vaccines with very little crossover market—they recently applied to the EMA for regulatory approval of their malaria vaccine, RTS,S, for example. Like most efforts in the private sector, however, GSK does not take its vaccine candidates all the way to market without subsidization. GSK thus partnered with Aeras to help finance and conduct a Phase IIb trial currently enrolling HIV-negative adults with latent tuberculosis in South Africa, Kenya, and Zambia. The aim is to enroll 3,500 participants with a thirty-six month follow-up and results by 2018 (Aeras 2014). Despite requiring assistance with the efficacy trial, Voss was adamant about GSK's commitment to manufacturing the vaccine and distributing it worldwide should it prove marketable (personal communication, July 6, 2012).

Discussions concerning collaborative imperatives for tuberculosis vaccine production have been underway for some time under the aegis of Aeras, the Stop TB Partnership Working Group on Vaccines, the WHO, the NIH, the National Institute of Allergy and Infectious Diseases (NIAID), BMGF, and TBVI, and involving academic, regulatory, nonprofit, private, and philanthropic sectors of vaccine research and development. That these conversations are happening on an occasional but regular basis across so many constituencies is rare in itself, suggesting not just a potential but at least in part a realization of changed rules of therapeutic production. Discussions so far have emphasized the need to share information with every stakeholder on the status of TB vaccine development, the scientific challenges being encountered, and the areas of research needing prioritization. Implicit in this agenda is a departure from proprietary norms within the private pharmaceutical sector that preclude sharing of information regarding product development and that impede productive conversations with multiple constituencies about logistical or scientific barriers to vaccine development. These discussions, in turn, were published by Michael Brennan of Aeras and Jelle Thole of TBVI, as an industry-wide blueprint for tuberculosis vaccine development (Brennan and Thole 2012).

In addition to articulating the critical nature of information sharing across scientific disciplines and industry sectors, Brennan and Thole actually go further in suggesting the need to reach across disease fields in efforts to gain scientific knowledge and experience necessary for TB vaccine work. Acknowledging the productive potential of scientific failure, Brennan and Thole call for publishing and sharing data on the clinical failures of malaria, HIV, and cancer as well as TB vaccine candidates given the important lessons to be learned from why vaccines fail at various stages of development (2012, S12). They also call for what they suggest is "creativity in research and development" of TB vaccines given the "profound" lack of knowledge of what constitutes protective immunity against TB in different age groups and populations, and given the critical knowledge missing from the arenas of immunology, microbiology, pathology, molecular biology, and vaccinology (Brennan and Thole 2012, S7).

This innovation is already beginning to happen. The failure of MVA85A and other vaccine research is generating insights into, and more focus on, harmonizing animal and human experiments, improving predictiveness of animal models, and replacing the latent/active binaries with the concept of a spectrum of disease (Frick 2014). Elaborating on the animal model problem, some pathogens act at the cellular level in particular animals much the way they would in humans, but this is not true of *M. tuberculosis*. Animal studies are still done, but they are too often not especially predictive of success in human trials. This, in turn, means spending time and money enrolling individuals in human trials that are doomed to fail.

In addition to the first trial combining two vaccine candidates, Aeras is also planning an innovation in their trial with GSK's M72 by collecting samples as part of a parallel study to look for correlates of protection from disease (Frick 2014). In another Phase II trial, Aeras is initiating a novel clinical trial design that will test another vaccine candidate, H4 + IC31, for its ability to prevent infection rather than disease. As stated in Aeras's press release, this change means being able to design a trial that enrolls fewer individuals and that is able to end more quickly because infection with *M. tuberculosis* can be detected almost immediately, rather than waiting for the onset of clinical symptoms as the trial endpoint.

The authors of the blueprint, not to mention the TB vaccine network, also recognize the need to go beyond information sharing to brokering more partnerships in efforts to expedite progress of vaccine development (Brennan and Thole 2012, S12). How to forge partnerships with "productive friction," and with whom, has become especially trenchant with recent industry exits from the field of tuberculosis research and development. This includes not just large pharmaceutical companies but smaller biotech firms such as Emergent BioSolutions, who announced soon after the failure of the MVA85A infant trial that there was no commercial market for a tuberculosis vaccine and that consequently they were closing their UK offices (Lockhart 2013). Precariousness extends then not just to how Aeras and TB Alliance nurture and navigate collaborations, but how they actually achieve them in a sustained way. When I asked Tom Evans, then CEO of Aeras, about the nature of collaborations and what he looks for in forging them, his responses were insightful and not limited to vaccines.

Science, Markets, and Learning Curves

First of all, as Evans immediately stated, the nature of the collaboration depends on the stage of development. In the early phases, what Aeras cares most about is the science, the quality of the investigators, and the integrity of the data. By Phase II trials, there is a gradual change from an emphasis on collaborative scientific research to more organizational structure including reasonable scientific, legal, and licensing departments. Academic partners or biotech firms typify collaborators at these stages. By Phase IIb, however, they begin looking for a competent larger partner, namely a pharmaceutical company with organizational as well as manufacturing skills. Yet, as Evans notes, the "organizational magnitude, commercial viability, regulatory expertise, and ability to roll out operations in multiple places in the world"—in other words, the facets needed for widespread deployment of a vaccine—discounts even many industry players. "Of the twenty [pharmaceutical companies] who think they have this [capability]," he noted drily, "only about ten really do." The question, of course, then becomes whether industry players want to get involved in pharmaceutical humanitarianism, and if so, how. The "why" is less concerning to Evans. As he notes, "if pharmaceutical companies have the mission to save the world and at the same time make some money, they [Aeras] are fine with that; or if they want to win the Nobel Prize, they are fine with that; or make a [vaccine] platform and then sell their company, they are fine with that—as long as they are also aligned with making a TB vaccine to save the world" (personal communication, January 26, 2012).

Ann Ginsberg, now the chief medical officer of Aeras, put it somewhat differently when saying that no matter how important something might be, if it isn't going to get you the product, it can't be pursued (personal communication, December 6, 2011). She was referring to the critical function of the private sector in late-stage vaccine development and the importance of finding out ways to arrive at "win-win contractual relationships." Key to this process is the fact that several individuals at Aeras, including Evans, Ginsberg, and Connolly, have come from business or private pharmaceutical companies and therefore understand the particular kinds of pressures characterizing those from the private sector, what their competing priorities might be, and the challenges they contend with if they become involved in nonlucrative areas of research and development. They have a better understanding, then, of what will motivate individuals from pharmaceutical companies to form collaborations with PDPs such as Aeras (Ginsberg, personal communication, December 6, 2011). As Joao Biehl puts it in describing the ascendancy of PDPs in global health, "Whatever differences there are across corporate, activist, and public health agendas the new rubric of 'value' appears to reconcile these differences and folds them into an ethos of collective responsibility" (2011, 106).

What constitutes "value" might be very different for industry players, but its pursuit can lead—however temporarily—to the same goal. Evans elaborated on this point, saying that the strategy at Aeras is always to "be proactive in that when the crack opens, they try to expand it; but they don't force a crack where there is none" (personal communication, January 26, 2011). Yet partnership forging is not unilateral—almost every major pharmaceutical company had thought about collaborations with a PDP like Aeras and inquired what a partnership would involve (Evans, personal communication, January 26, 2011). This mutual dependency exemplifies less a melding of values as a forging of humanitarian and CSR interests that prove mutually beneficial as long as the end goals do not conflict.

Indeed both Evans and Ginsberg—like their TB Alliance counterparts—made abundantly clear to me the highly varied and even unpredictable motivations behind industry involvement in partnerships for tuberculosis vaccines. Assuming that the pharmaceutical industry is just engaging in PDPs to repair bad public relations without actually doing anything substantive is not always inaccurate, yet it is overly simplistic. Many pharmaceutical companies involved in PDPs do have motivations anchored in CSR, but some are redirecting their visions of commercial potential at the same time, namely aiming at what is being called the bottom-of-the-pyramid (BOP), high-volume, low-cost market model encompassing the millions of low-income but high-disease-burden populations globally (Prahalad and Hart 2002). Profits in the BOP model will not match those from the blockbuster era given how low prices would likely need to be. Yet there are also ample middle classes in India, China, South Africa, and Brazil who will need tuberculosis vaccines, and this of course is also something of which pharmaceutical companies are aware.

Corporations would likely not stop at tuberculosis vaccines, however. As Ginsberg suggests, once actively established in these markets, pharmaceutical companies can begin turning their attention toward therapeutics aimed at cancers or at chronic diseases like hypertension, both of which afflict ever-increasing numbers in BRICS countries. As she added, there is obvious business sense in building relationships with the "really big markets" in countries like China, India, or Brazil. This is particularly appealing for pharmaceutical companies in the UK, EU, or United States where there is widespread saturation in home markets and where large middle classes in other countries are needed to revitalize slumping drug sales. Working first on a high-priority public health disease like tuberculosis gains them a "halo effect"—that is, it goes some distance in countering the widespread criticism of pharmaceutical companies that profit rather than health is their only bottom line. If they are making earnest efforts to codevelop tuberculosis vaccines within the country, they are showing they have good intent and diversified motivations. Using tuberculosis vaccines as an entrée into BRICS countries also teaches each pharmaceutical company how to work in these new markets without at first necessarily having pressures of simultaneously making a profit. If they become the first pharmaceutical company in fifty years to license a new TB vaccine or drug, the halo effect will help them gain trust while they learn to negotiate regulatory and other regional structures. Tuberculosis, then, becomes a learning curve for pharmaceutical companies in new markets (Ginsberg, personal communication, December 6, 2011).

Evans and Ginsberg also mentioned other motivations underlying industry decisions to expand into tuberculosis research, such as better science or opportunities to do proof of concept (Phase IIb) studies. And, importantly, beneath the broader company-level agendas are the scientists working for these companies "for the right reasons," that is, because they want to make a difference. Drawing on her time at Merck as well as at Aeras and TB Alliance, Ginsberg suggested that "both at the highest level in some cases, and with all companies at project team level, there are people really jazzed at working on such a huge urgent medical need. . . . It excites them to get out of bed and know they are helping the millions of TB patients around the world, instead of working to develop another me-too drug" (personal communication, December 6, 2011).

Like TB Alliance, Aeras approached China as a potentially key partner in their mission, recently signing an agreement for TB vaccine research and development with the Chinese biotechnology company China National Biotech Group (Aeras 2012b). The reasons for this move are multiple and mutually reinforcing, with the definition of "value" overlapping with, yet ultimately diverging from, that of industry. Aeras recognizes what TB Alliance did, namely that China has a high tuberculosis burden coupled with ample financial resources and an already well-developed pharmaceutical and scientific sector. And importantly, tuberculosis is a priority for the Chinese government (Ginsberg, personal communication, December 6, 2011). From the funding standpoint, China becomes a partner in furthering Aeras's agenda by potentially financing a significant proportion of research and development of vaccine candidates including late-stage clinical trials and manufacturing—facets that Aeras would otherwise have to pay for (Ginsberg, personal communication, December 6, 2011). But China's arena of scientific expertise and infrastructure specifically related to tuberculosis is less robust, so they in turn will be the beneficiary of technology and knowledge transfer from Aeras (Evans, personal communication, January 26, 2011). So China receives assistance in producing vaccines for the large number of Chinese at risk of tuberculosis while also enhancing their scientific and biopharmaceutical capabilities. As noted by Evans, beyond developing vaccines for domestic consumption, China eventually could assume a leadership position in exporting vaccines to the rest of the world given its inherent capabilities (personal communication, January 26, 2011).

This last comment is a reminder that pharmaceutical and biotechnical development is playing a strategic role in China's economic development, as it has in many parts of the world (see Ong and Chen 2010; Jeong 2013). But as Aihwa Ong in particular has noted, the role of biotechnological development goes beyond the economy, extending to the expansion of national visibility and regional and global power. It responds as well to recent biosecurity threats from infectious disease outbreaks such as SARS and influenza, providing a space for stronger state response in tandem with building scientific expertise and infrastructure to ensure better and faster regional response to outbreaks. After SARS and H1N1 there was a reaction throughout regions of Asia more generally against Western imaginaries of Asia as a hotspot of infectious disease (MacPhail 2014). There was also a growing perception that pharmaceutical research was dominated by Westerners and that Asian scientists needed to work on diseases affecting Asian populations and from an Asian perspective (Ong 2010; MacPhail 2014). TB Alliance and Aeras thus clearly are also playing a symbolic and strategic development role with their participation in China's pharmaceutical and biotechnology sector buildup by working closely with the government and by specifically addressing a disease of significant impact within China. Here, Chinese technical, state, and scientific sectors converge with PDP expertise to form an alternative and more geopolitically equitable version of humanitarian pharmaceutical production, one that by default will incorporate Asian expertise and localized perspective.

Geographies and Scales of Finance

Geography clearly has become prominent in how PDPs see the road ahead, but it is not a particularly straight road. As noted by Mel Spigelman of TB Alliance, China represents something of a game changer in PDPs. It is not just that China possesses huge resources and an equally huge population in need of TB drugs or vaccines; it is that they do business differently. Nonprofits are not the only ones starting to do business with Chinese biotechs and pharmaceutical companies—there is "huge interest" among pharmaceutical companies in forging partnerships with the Chinese pharmaceutical sector. And both have to work the way Chinese companies and, de facto, the Chinese government work, not the way they are used to working. A different form of capitalism clearly inheres in how China does business, including how it produces pharmaceuticals.

There is, for example, a much closer relationship between government and industry in China, and all potential partners have to be cognizant of that if collaborations are going to work. As an example, Spigelman noted that universal access for China is not synonymous with not-for-profit. "China provides TB drugs to all of its population right now. . . . But that doesn't mean that Chinese manufacturers are pro bono; they are making a profit" (personal communication, December 7, 2011). They make a profit, but they work within the regulatory and financial directives of the government.

BRICS countries, but China in particular, thus hold a potentially key place not just in the partnerships Aeras and TB Alliance form, but in their changing financial configurations. For both TB Alliance and Aeras, China in particular represents one way to wean off of the current reliance on BMGF and other soft money that will not remain available forever, and that in effect keeps PDPs in a persistent state of financial precariousness and contingency. The arrangements being brokered by both organizations are beneficial to China and its goal to strengthen its pharmaceutical sector, diminish tuberculosis, and "figure out how to globalize" as Spigelman put it (personal communication, December 7, 2011). While doing this, however, PDPs hope that China will benefit them by paying for a significant portion of the costs of developing vaccines and drug regimens. What this means for how drug and vaccine production might potentially change given China's variant mode of government-regulated, public health–oriented capitalism is hard to answer given the nascent state of collaborations, but Spigelman in particular suggests it will be something to watch given China's critical role within Asia and beyond.

At the same time, Spigelman suggested that PDPs might be following pharmaceutical partners in shifting their focus to chronic diseases five years down the road—a point that I found startling given the foundational missions of both Aeras and TB Alliance. As he asked, is there something to be learned in the PDP model that is transferable to chronic diseases as their treatment becomes mandated in the developing world? (personal communication, December 7, 2011). Clearly the answer is "yes." On March 11, 2014, TB Alliance announced that it was assigning its patents on "bi-functional compounds" to a Chinese-based biotech company, TenNor. These compounds were produced in the process of tuberculosis drug research and development, but instead of proving effective in treating tuberculosis they were found more suitable for bacterially caused gastrointestinal diseases. TenNor will develop the compounds for these gastrointestinal indications, and the proceeds from their hoped-for sales down the road will be put back into tuberculosis drug development (TB Alliance 2014a). Chinese biotechs like TenNor, and the wealth of diseases to treat in China's huge population, are thus adding further dimensions to the critical role of BRICS countries in PDP sustainability. This particular example also suggests the symbiotic relationship of diverse infectious diseases in PDP financial models, just as the role of malaria did in PDP research models. It also possibly portends the expansion of PDP remit from treating only those infectious diseases designated by BMGF and other donors, to treating a broader array of infectious and even possibly chronic diseases.

Innovative financing like this is another arena indicating how PDPs are coming to terms with the need to branch out beyond BMGF and government donations. That the BMGF has been a major force in both organizations' operations is incontestable, with virtually every individual remarking to me that the degree to which tuberculosis PDPs have accomplished as much as they have in the last ten years is due to BMGF largesse. Yet everyone is equally aware that this largesse cannot last for long, nor is it without parameters. Though everyone spoke in positive terms about BMGF donations (how could they not), it is clear that there are particular kinds of initiatives that BMGF is willing to fund and particular criteria used for determining what is and is not targeted for resource allocations. For example, the foundation is less willing to fund initiatives like developing clinical trial sites because, though critical to moving promising drugs or vaccines further down the pipeline, trial site capacity-building itself produces little to show in terms of lives saved, disease rates diminished, or numbers of drugs or vaccines dispersed. It exemplifies the point made in the previous chapter, that an emphasis on statistics and measurable outcomes is indicative of what many current foundations including the BMGF are looking for (Yanacopulos 2011; Bull and McNeill 2007).

Regardless of the current parameters, the need for other and more sustainable sources of funding has been growing as PDPs have matured. That search includes finding financing mechanisms that are derivative of the private sector yet tweaked to fit the fundamental mission of affordability and accessibility to all regions in need of tuberculosis therapeutics. As indicated by Kari Stoever, Aeras's former vice president of external affairs, she saw her role at Aeras as, among other things, framing TB in a way that helps investors understand the nature and magnitude of the problem, but also in thinking about nontraditional ways of developing IP. While illustrating her ideas via a PowerPoint slide, she talked about the way in which science and financing "come into the portfolio, together," one opening possibilities for the other and vice versa. At the very beginning stages of research, for example, grant money is the most likely source of funding because not enough is known about any new product to attract venture capital. The more we know about tuberculosis vaccines and their protective mechanisms, the more assurances investors have that they are "picking the right horse in the race" (personal communication, June 6, 2012).

Picking the right horse is easier at later stages given the scientific certainties gained from early-stage clinical trials. Yet more robust knowledge comes with more robust price tags, and hence the "Valley of Death" moniker—that is, the inevitable paucity of funding for later, more expensive stages of clinical research. This is where Stoever has tried several financing options, including being more creative with European and Asian development banks that have more of a social mission and for whom lower returns on investment are more acceptable.[6] As Stoever indicated, being able to get even some returns on debt or investment is just starting to happen. Or, it might be possible to devise "payback clauses" in IP agreements where the (U.S.) government would pay back the bank loan if the product fails, but commercial manufacturers would pay it back through royalty schemes if it succeeds. Stoever suggested the possibility of creating a new, for-profit organization that could negotiate IP agreements with access provisions still included, but also a payback clause upon the success of the vaccine candidate. Licensing or selling IP to big pharma also would help recoup money not just for paying back loans but for further investment into more R&D—what TB Alliance did with TenNor but scaled up. But, Stoever insisted, it would still be a PDP model, still a partnership. As she put it, Aeras still has to de-risk PDP endeavors for pharma, but using finance and capital more creatively they can do this while also sustaining their portfolio (personal communication, June 6, 2012).

Indeed, in Aeras and TBVI's document written for prospective investors (Stoever and Thole 2013), rigorous management of their portfolio, among other things, is critical to the argument for increased investment from the private sector. The document is a unique blend of standard financial arguments, epidemiologic explanation, and humanitarian appeal. Detailing the global scourge of a preventable disease sets the stage for humanitarian investment opportunities topped with moral politics, followed by an assurance of eventual returns on investment: the "initial market assessments" indicate that the first ten years of commercializing at low cost a tuberculosis vaccine targeting adolescents and adults could generate revenue in the $12–13 billion range. The research and development pipeline becomes a "value chain" with "push mechanisms" like grants taking care of most costs for early-stage research. What Aeras needs are "pull mechanisms" like blended capital "utilizing debt and/or equity" that can leverage what attenuated pharmaceutical involvement remains at the late stages of clinical research (Stoever and Thole 2013).

The meticulous outline of how every candidate in the portfolio is subject to standardized financial and scientific criteria joins the other elements of this report to present to banks and private investors a multilateral argument for financial support, couched in language that investors listen to—including language that minimizes risk. This is a savvy document that speaks to the maturation of a nonprofit organization understanding that its ideals of pharmaceutical humanitarianism and the innovative financial, scientific, and collaborative architectures it produces nevertheless do not exist outside the overarching imperative of capital. The point where humanitarianism in pharmaceutical production meets capital will remain uneasy, given that this juncture epitomizes the contradiction of the humanitarian ideal with the insurmountable expense of achieving the desired end results. Tuberculosis PDPs then have to find a way to incorporate financial mechanisms posing the least threat to the integrity of its ideological and technical architecture. This juncture also evidences what almost everyone I spoke with reminded me in the early stages of my research when I referred to Aeras's and TB Alliance's work as nonprofit. "It is not nonprofit, it is low profit" was the admonition I got, indicating the realization from the beginning of these organizations that even a low level of profit would aid their own operations with reinvestment into research, but also signal to industry that at least some profit was a part of the multiple dimensions of value encompassed within their endeavor.

Conclusion

Risk mitigation as a necessary prerequisite for gaining industry participation in PDP efforts is a point I heard repeatedly in conversations and at conferences. It exists uneasily alongside the enthusiasm I witnessed from more than one pharmaceutical scientist heading their company's version of an infectious disease or access-to-medicines department. Though receiving resource allocations from their parent companies worth only a fraction of those dedicated to more traditional treatments and their respective markets, these initiatives are not negligible: the few companies remaining in the game continue to make strides in developing promising products and are taken very seriously by the scientists heading them. They also go beyond many initiatives more clearly residing within the heading of CSR.

To the extent that pharmaceutical companies participating in tuberculosis PDPs do so primarily as CSR, this needs more discussion. There is no question that some CSR actions can be beneficial, such as medicine donation programs that succeed in diminishing well-entrenched infectious diseases. At the same time, much of pharmaceutical company CSR has been criticized for doing more for public relations than disease mitigation and, in some instances, for using actions like drug donations as a tool to undermine locally produced generics (Ecks 2008). Seeing these initiatives only within the frame of global corporate citizenship, however, automatically exposes them to the more damning critique of enhancing global public relations rather than making serious attempts at ameliorating burdens of disease—confining these efforts, that is, to the ostensibly irreconcilable poles of making profit versus acting ethically. As the anthropologist Stefan Ecks concludes, "global corporate citizenship is not a brake on free-wheeling capitalism, but rather a strategy of extending and accelerating it by new means" (2008, 178).

Ecks means this as an accusation of pharmaceutical companies' duplicity in passing drug donations off as a form of pastoral care rather than underhanded profit-making, and his case study of Novartis and their drug Gleevac in India certainly supports this. Without detracting from his claims, I want to suggest that the seemingly contradictory goals of ethical action and profit incentive are not mutually exclusive. Those leading the corporate TB drug and vaccine R&D initiatives are doing exactly what Ecks goes on to suggest, namely that "it would be more ethical by corporations to tone down the claim of being a 'good citizen' and to state in simple capitalist terms why they are doing what they are doing" (2008, 178). Those with whom I spoke from the corporate sector openly discussed the short- and long-term marketing benefits of tuberculosis initiatives, but also talked about the imbrication—not contradiction—of new market strategies with social missions to better address diseases of poverty. And to rephrase what the head of one pharmaceutical's infectious diseases department said, their work on infectious diseases is part good will gesture and part response to the disciplining condemnation of global public opinion. It is sadly ironic that pharmaceutical companies might now profit socially if not financially from the disease burdens they helped create through their own strident pursuit of pharmaceuticals with hefty financial returns to the neglect of public health. Dealing with that irony, however, is better than industry continuing the status quo of the last decades or ignoring the equally strident public condemnation of pharmaceutical practices and the calls to redress the neglect.

Highly dubious ethics continue to characterize some mainstream pharmaceutical practices, however, and thus the larger but largely unanswerable question remains of how pharmaceutical companies themselves see the relationship between their efforts in infectious disease research and the rest of what they do. Obviously, as seen in persistent lawsuits, criminal indictments, and claims of malfeasance, the former does not absolve the latter nor should it. But focusing on the initiatives of companies like Sanofi and GSK in tuberculosis research, the more pressing question in the short term remains what the new forms of financial and social value are going to look like in humanitarian pharmaceutical production. The increasing sophistication of Aeras and TB Alliance in tapping the multiplicity of pharmaceutical motivations for getting involved in tuberculosis research, and finding increasingly innovative means of de-risking that participation, provides some optimism. But the very *fact* of having to de-risk points to a persistent stumbling block in these alternative formations of pharmaceutical production: how to reconcile the prohibitive expense of developing new tuberculosis drugs and vaccines with the prospects of a low return on investment; and related, how to effect a larger shift in how pharmaceutical companies approach relations of market, investment, and disease burdens so that de-risking is no longer a necessity in PDP practices. The partnerships with China recently forged by both Aeras and TB Alliance, the innovative financing described by Stoever, and the leveraging of TB research through (future) sales of gastrointestinal drugs are evident steps in this direction.

In the meantime, Tom Evans asked a question I was unprepared for. In my open-ended interviews, I always asked individuals if there were pertinent questions I had not raised. Evans's startling response to that was, "If you wanted a TB vaccine made for the world, is a PDP the best model to do it in?" And he followed up with declaring that subsidizing industry has not necessarily been a bad model, even if it is not as cost-effective or humanitarian (personal communication, January 26, 2011). It is certainly a fair question, even if from a surprising source. Yet in this case, the first response is the most obvious—that industry with few exceptions never had, or has, any intentions of producing a new tuberculosis vaccine on its own for the reasons already articulated. One thing about PDPs is abundantly clear, and that is that they are highly interdependent entities. Aeras can't make a vaccine without industry, but the opposite is equally true.

The second response is embedded within Evans's qualifier—that is, to the extent that pharmaceutical companies do produce vaccines for all kinds of infectious diseases, and to the extent that they have been doing so collaboratively, this does not make them humanitarian given their record on equity in access and distribution. Influenza vaccines are a good case in point: during the 2009 H1N1 outbreak, not only were few pharmaceutical companies willing to take on the liability of producing a vaccine, but they distributed the vaccines they did produce first to the populations in their home countries, and then to those governments such as the United States and EU who possessed the financial means to precontract doses for their own populations. Low-income countries finally got vaccine shipments only after the United States and a few European countries donated their leftover vaccines—only enough to cover a negligible fraction of any country's population, and only long after the peak of the epidemic was over. Had the outbreak been as virulent as initially feared, fatalities would have been grossly uneven yet predictable in their geographic distribution (Craddock and Giles-Vernick 2010).

The answer to Evans's question, then, gets to the heart of why PDPs are so necessary, at least in the current historical moment. It is not just about efficiency or even about collaboration by itself. Those traits only become something politically galvanizing when they are tethered to notions of equitable access across all geographies, and when disease burdens gain a prominent place in determining biotechnological research and development directives. PDPs focused on addressing infectious diseases including tuberculosis are some of the few entities currently attempting to operationalize a huge shift in current norms and apparatuses of pharmaceutical production. The adroitness characterizing PDPs such as those TB Alliance and Aeras are spearheading is a strength in these efforts; it allows for some unprecedented interventions into the very ontological foundations of pharmaceutical production: of what and how pharmaceutical products are made, and for whom. The partnerships they forge manage to be productive even in their highly dynamic and sometimes tentative, divergent, and even contradictory motivations.

As will be taken up in the next chapter, PDPs' innovation continues in their scientific practices, at the same time that the nature of tuberculosis itself, coupled with inadequate knowledge of how it acts in the body, means that the expense of developing tuberculosis therapies is higher than average. Prohibitive expense, in turn, can threaten the parameters of low-profit innovation since it drives the need for more conventional sources of capital, which in turn threatens the very meaning and integrity of the PDP concept and the model of hybridity they have achieved. Even as I was impressed by the innovative financing schemes described by Stoever, I wondered whether the necessity of drawing increasingly on investments from the private sector was the brilliant antidote to donor dependency, while simultaneously the beginning of a slippery slope away from the founding missions of these endeavors. Either way it makes clear that the impossibility, so far, for PDPs to disentangle themselves from a larger world of low-risk, high-profit investment decisions creates both possibilities and contradictions in how they can accomplish their goals, and whether it will drive a change in those goals even in the near future. Ironically, it is advances in tuberculosis research that might answer this conundrum.

2 SCIENTIFIC COLLABORATION, INNOVATION, AND CONTRADICTION

THE INNOVATIONS TUBERCULOSIS PDPs MAKE do not stop at their partnerships and financing mechanisms. They encompass scientific practices, knowledge sharing, and regulatory policies, to name a few, informed by an overarching belief in the social value of what they do. From these multiple arenas of conduct, fields of value are created that extend well beyond, yet encompass, the products they are developing. But before elaborating on these innovations for TB Alliance, Aeras, and their collaborators, the contrasting definition of innovation within the commercial pharmaceutical sector is helpful.

The problem is that the definition of innovation within the industry is not obvious. In the last few years there has been an increasing chorus of analysts concerned with what appears to be an overall decline in pharmaceutical innovation over the last several decades. The argument and the statistics to back it up are variably expressed. A recent Government Accounting Office report, for example, cites a 40 percent decline in New Drug Applications (NDAs) to the FDA between 1995 and 2004 despite an increase of money going into drug research (GAO 2007, 3). Another study by David Horrobin claims a drop in new chemical entity (NCE) applications from an average industry-wide yearly output of eighty to one hundred in the 1960s to only thirty to forty in the late 1990s (2000).[1] Yet another study by an insider to industry, Bernard Munos of Eli Lilly, shows that new molecular entity (NME) approvals have remained constant since 1950, not declined;[2] yet given that financial resources channeled into drug development have risen exponentially over the same time period, a flat rate of output is concerning (2009).

On the surface, this concern is appropriate: certainly in the United

States we have come to expect pharmaceuticals to improve well-being, prolong life, and combat chronic and degenerative diseases. We also presume that drugs and vaccines will be developed to target new diseases such as SARS or HIV when they emerge. But the discussions surrounding the concern, and the flatlining of pharmaceutical innovation, are themselves instructive. Though some disease-specific studies cite the need for greater innovation in drug development to prolong the lives of those with cancer, for example, the majority of studies discussing drug innovation do so with no mention of patients or the enhanced well-being of particular populations. Instead, concern over innovation is discussed within the context of declining profit: innovation is an engine of financial health for the pharmaceutical industry, not for individuals or populations. NCEs or NMEs or drug applications are appraised not as to how many people's lives will be improved, but how much return on investments they are predicted to generate. As Donald Light and Joel Lexchin suggest, the real crisis in innovation comes not in the low number of NMEs approved by the FDA per se, but in the low number that actually represent a therapeutic advance rather than yet another of several similar drugs basically doing the same thing (2012).

Innovation, in other words, has become virtually synonymous with profit generation within the pharmaceutical industry. Pharmaceutical research and development have been naturalized to a definition resting upon the number of NMEs or NCEs promising high financial returns and, as such, have generated their own particular legal, practical, and procedural mechanisms for improving innovation so defined. These include metrics, timelines, and priorities for how research is done within pharmaceutical companies, as well as mergers, "me-too" drugs, the practice of extending patents called "ever-greening,"[3] and industry litigation in cases of patent encroachment to name a few. None of these has much to do with what should be the more obvious imperative of pharmaceutical innovation—that is, saving lives and improving health. As another industry insider recently put it, his five decades within the pharmaceutical industry showed him that "the primary goal of research changed from discovery and social usefulness to making money" (Firestone 2011).

None of this is surprising in the sense that the pharmaceutical industry is one among many answering to their shareholders and exercising the parameters of contemporary global capitalist practices focused on quarterly profits and lower expenditures. Except, as Firestone goes on to suggest, today's ruling corporate philosophy of micromanagement, time lines, and efficiency is "suited to selling automobiles" rather than pharmaceutical products. Generating innovation within the pharmaceutical industry, Firestone claims—and by this, he means actually making new and socially useful discoveries and producing new products—requires time for contemplation and intuitive leaps (2011). As Munos similarly admits, when lags in pharmaceutical innovation happen in the midst of a "golden age of scientific discovery," the current corporate research and development model emphasizing short-term priorities and reliable returns on investment needs to be rethought. Yet rather than overturn industry R&D practices, he tellingly suggests that breakthrough discoveries will only happen outside of corporate walls, where scientific thinking and doing beyond "the pressures of market needs" can be allowed to lead to what he calls "disruptive innovation." He mentions public–private partnerships, among other entities, as examples of "radical and successful experiments" where innovation is actually happening (Munos 2009, 966).

It is a very candid admission that creative and exciting research cannot happen within a corporate model, yet it is apparently in agreement with 360 other pharmaceutical executives who predicted in a 2008 survey that most research and development in the next decade would happen outside of large life science companies (cited in Sunder Rajan 2012, 323). As Sunder Rajan points out in an article evaluating the political economics and value logics of therapeutic production, developing effective therapeutics is part of a "structure of contradiction" because producing therapeutics is what pharmaceutical companies do, yet when therapies are effective people stop taking them because they feel better. In other words, "the pharmaceutical industry is rare in that its products, if they work, obviate their own necessity" (2012, 329).[4] But exacerbating the contradiction, as Sunder Rajan goes on to explain, is the location of most large pharmaceutical companies in a speculative, shareholder-driven marketplace that demands consistent market growth at rates that cannot be met through development of therapeutic compounds alone. Hence, the turn toward mergers and acquisitions, ever-greening, and off-label uses of drugs. For wealthier markets, there is also the shift from therapeutics aimed at improving diseased states to those enhancing healthy states or mitigating future decline: what Joseph Dumit calls the cultivation of surplus health or Sunder Rajan designates as "economies of therapeutic excess and saturation" (Dumit 2012; Sunder Rajan 2012, 337).

In contrast, TB Alliance, Aeras, and their collaborators are configuring innovation to a set of expectations, agendas, creativities, and protocols aimed at social usefulness and the health of populations, rather than the health of corporations or their shareholders. The products Aeras and TB Alliance are aiming to develop are those that, as Ann Ginsberg put it, "would make the biggest difference to the most people" (personal communication, December 6, 2011): in other words, they would be delivered to as many people as possible who are at risk of, or already suffer from, tuberculosis. For tuberculosis PDPs, producing effective therapeutics that obviate their own necessity is the ultimate mark of their success, not an economic contradiction. As such, they are regalvanizing the value of time, failure, collaboration, and knowledge sharing in their development of new therapeutic technologies, and in so doing illustrating that these technologies are inextricable from the relations that constitute them.

Andrew Barry, in his work on the making of the molecule, suggests that molecular compounds are not just a combination of atoms or molecules but rather are constituted in their relations to informational and material environments (2005, 52, 56). Drawing from the science studies scholars Bernadette Bensaude-Vincent and Isabel Stengers, Barry argues that a range of information including data on potency, dosing, and toxicity, clinical trial results, IP regimes, and regulatory approvals actually enters into and makes compounds what they are, how they are perceived, and how they are acted upon. Newer research methods according to Barry take drug discovery from "craft laboratory skills" to industrialized methods, while also imbuing substantial social and scientific, if not economic, capital in the results. These newer methods include combinatorial chemistry, where large numbers of molecules can be generated from smaller molecular fragments and combined in different sets and sequences,[5] and high-throughput screening, enabling scientists to test hundreds of thousands of compounds against particular "targets" (like *M. tuberculosis*) to see if they seem promising (Barry 2005).

Scientific practices involved in producing tuberculosis compounds and vaccine candidates constitute, and are constituted by, similar information on dosing, safety data, stability, and regulatory status, among other legal and material environments. Much of this kind of information is globally regulated—part of a standardization of scientific practices instituted through the International Conference on Harmonization (ICH) in 1990, and intended to make clinical research and pharmaceutical manufacturing adhere to the same safety and ethics standards no matter where in the world they are conducted. These requirements extend to good clinical practices (GCP), good manufacturing practices (GMP), and good laboratory practices (GLP) in the research and development of new pharmaceuticals. Conforming to the rules of each of these is required for FDA or EMA approval. But in addition to these standard practices, PDPs create their own environments based on exigencies and circumstances peculiar to their humanitarian approaches. Equally important for them, for example, is the information derived from their attention to conditions pertaining in regions slated for new pharmaceuticals, alternative propri-etary arrangements, and expanded spaces for knowledge sharing in the research and development process. Also unavoidable for them, however, are the parameters of industrial commitments and behavior of the bac-terium itself as well as the limits of scientific knowledge about it. All of these fields of desire, contingency, and action make the molecular com-pounds and vaccine candidates at the center of PDP efforts distinctly constituted and valued. In the rest of the chapter I elaborate on these fields and how they contour humanitarian pharmaceutical production.

Revaluing Failure

I did not know exactly what to expect when I arrived in Rockville, outside of Washington, D.C., to take a tour of Aeras's vaccine production plant. Jamie Rosen, the former media and communications manager for Aeras, had explained to me that the plant was the facility for Aeras's scientists to conduct their research, but also a manufacturing plant that allowed them to save money by keeping that facet of research, testing, and rollout in-house. What I found was a sleek new red brick building that could have been the corporate headquarters of any midsize company in the United States. And the plant was seamlessly incorporated next to Aeras's offices, enabling a greater degree of communication and traffic between research-ers and other employees. Indeed, heads of research units could have meetings with science officers or marketing directors and then go back to the research and manufacturing facility for immediate communication and input to the other researchers, ensuring a level of daily cross-communication that in some pharmaceutical facilities would only hap-pen through telecommunications.

David McCown, Aeras's affable senior manager overseeing scientific progress, gave me a tour of the vaccine production facilities. While show-ing me some of the state-of-the-art vaccine development labs, McCown enthusiastically discussed the positive role of failure as well as creative thinking among the scientists. By this he meant precisely what Munos admitted was missing in his overview of pharmaceutical innovation in the commercial sector. As McCown implicitly recognizes, allowing a degree of creativity in the scientific process means by default leaving more latitude for failure. "Failure" of course holds a prominent and variable place in the history of science. Failures in particular designs—whether of bridges or of medical devices—can lend critical insights to improved designs in the future (see Petroski 2006); many current pharmaceuticals in use today failed at what they were originally designed to treat but ended up being effective in treating something else; or, of course, there is the oft-cited statistic that nine in ten compounds coming down the research and development pipeline will fail, usually in early clinical trials. Rather than an objective determination of loss, then, failure more often has been a flexible, context-driven part of always iterative and often unpredictable scientific processes.

In recent years, however, failure has largely come to possess negative connotations in the commercial pharmaceutical sector: with the increasing imbrication of innovation with profit, failure has come to signify a waste of time and, more importantly, a waste of financial investment. As pointed out by Dr. Carl Nathan of the Weill Cornell Medical College, the psychology behind industry decisions on what does or does not move forward in the pipeline is to drop whatever is not moving fast enough. This in turn means focusing on what is easier to develop by virtue of being familiar: rather than developing a new therapeutic, it is easier to take something that's been done before and do something slightly different with it (personal communication, July 31, 2014). This line of thinking drives me-too drugs or drugs for the same indication as many other drugs already on the market. The pressure to recoup millions of dollars when compounds do fail has also generated highly controversial practices in recent years among many large pharmaceutical companies, including shielding negative clinical trial results from publication and from the FDA so that drugs can proceed to market (see Healy 2006), or recontouring statistics to show apparent benefits of a new drug in subpopulations after trial results showed inadequate benefits in general populations (see Kahn 2012).

Seen against this recent configuration of failure, McCown's statement is more significant. To use Munos's phrase, "disruptive innovation" is happening at places like Aeras because failure is no longer a political or financial liability for scientists given leeway to try new things. In the process development phase, for example, the goal is to optimize the large-scale manufacturing potential of a vaccine candidate at the lowest cost possible in order to keep overall expenses down. Here, McCown encourages his researchers to think outside the box: to think creatively about how to accomplish the goal of scaling up vaccine candidate manufacturing while keeping costs as low as possible. What makes one candidate more expensive than another, according to McCown, is less often the expense of the materials that went into each vaccine, and more the methods and steps required in processing—that is, how much processing is needed, at what temperatures, how stable it is, and how many steps it takes to get a candidate ready for large-scale reproduction. Pointing to four small cylindrical bioreactors lined up along a wall of one unit, McCown indicated that batches are put in each cylinder and different processing approaches are taken with each—for example, slightly different angles of the paddles churning the liquid inside the cylinder, or changes in temperature. If or when a batch fails—that is, becomes unstable—they discard that, sanitize the cylinder, and start over. At this stage, as McCown said, failure was "just fine," a productive feature of the research process as it was instrumental in moving forward the equation of best quality at lowest manufacturing cost (personal communication, June 6, 2012).

Recalibrating Success

Just as failure is being brought back into the creative fold of science, what constitutes success within tuberculosis PDPs overlaps with, but also departs from, the commercial sector. For example, Ann Ginsberg noted that committees for deciding the criteria for which candidates are moved down the development pipeline are carefully chosen to represent various perspectives going well beyond anything commercial companies would be concerned about. So for both Aeras and TB Alliance, target product profiles, as these criteria are called, were informed by the scientific, business, and research communities, but they also included caregivers, national TB programs, ministries of health, and patient representatives: all of these have input as to what kinds of products each organization should be aiming for and what success should look like. Though this sometimes makes committee discussions "rich," as Ginsberg drily noted, it also signals an emphasis on maximizing breadth of consumption and its attendant impact on health, rather than on markets (personal communication, December 6, 2011).

A critical factor underlying these discussions is the more limited resources available to Aeras and TB Alliance relative to major pharmaceutical companies. This is why the "stage-gates" are important—that is, the criteria used to evaluate candidates at each stage of the development process and to make decisions on which candidates to move forward and which to shelve. Limited resources usually are associated with limited capacities to engage in broad-scale or cutting-edge research and development. Tom Evans put it in a more positive way when stating that more limited finances requires careful attention to prevent duplication of efforts and the advancement of multiple candidates with the same mechanism of action—practices common in the commercial sector (personal communication, January 26, 2012). Limited resources coupled with humanitarian ideals also mean honing the selection criteria to focus on the full "informational and material environments" of candidate drugs and vaccines, to use Barry's terms. Here, pharmaceuticals' research ecologies, their very meaning and litmus for success, is tied in with, inter alia, regional consumer preferences, public health impact, logistics of deployment, and challenges to national regulatory approval and adoption (Ginsberg, personal communication, December 6, 2011).

As to other specifics informing stage-gate decisions, one impediment can be when the IP practices of Aeras or TB Alliance collide with more typical commercial IP approaches. That is, sometimes Aeras or TB Alliance need to use a discovery patented by another pharmaceutical or biotech company in order to further their own candidates, but those companies are not willing to share. As Ginsberg put it, the question around IP is whether Aeras or others will have freedom to develop specific products for tuberculosis, or whether someone else can block their ability to do so because of patents on their discoveries (personal communication, December 6, 2011). For example, the research specialist Victor Prikhodko mentioned that Aeras was stymied in using adjuvants—components used in some vaccines to modulate immune-provoking capabilities—because most were patented by pharmaceutical companies unwilling to license them to Aeras at lower cost (personal communication, June 6, 2012). To elaborate, licensing costs—that is, what a patent owner charges for another agency to use their patented product—can play significantly into final costs of new vaccines and drugs, particularly in an age where patenting has increased as it has gone "upstream," that is, to ever earlier stages of research. Developing a new vaccine or drug can thus entail needing to license multiple components from other companies—from the duck cell lines mentioned in the previous chapter, to vaccine adjuvants, to delivery methods.

Pharmaceutical and biotech companies insisting on charging high fees for licensing their products can thus still exert influence over PDP research and development directions and the decisions they have to make on which candidates to move forward. How much the final product is going to cost is not surprisingly a major factor in decisions made by both Aeras and TB Alliance. Production cost is a starting point, as evidenced by McCown, but whether some drugs cost more because of an active ingredient, prohibitive licensing fees, or the manufacturing process, discussions can then focus on whether switching manufacturers, lowering doses, or other kinds of changes could reduce costs in a candidate otherwise showing promising trial results (Gardiner, personal communication, November 29, 2011).

Interestingly, on a tour of a GSK vaccine production facility outside of Brussels, I asked Gérald Voss, head of the unit that focuses on vaccines for neglected diseases, whether GSK took the same approach of having researchers find the lowest-cost candidates possible since these vaccines would overwhelmingly be destined for low-income countries. He looked a bit perplexed at this question before responding that no, what was most important was what works, not what was the least expensive. So, he went on, if the vaccine candidate that seemed the most efficacious is the most complex molecule that will thus be the most expensive to move forward, that's what you go with. "You want what is the most effective, and then you hope that countries can find a way to implement them, through purchasing organizations like GAVI[6] or UNICEF" (personal communication, July 6, 2012). In other words, GSK does not internalize responsibility for balancing the best science and evidence of efficacy with the means available to lessen costs to eventual consumers. They externalize cost issues to global purchasing organizations, despite these organizations' variable funding levels and consequent capacity to cover all needed vaccines for all low-income countries. It perhaps raises a question about Voss's claim that GSK is dedicated to making sure their tuberculosis vaccine candidate, M72, gets to those who need it should it prove efficacious.

Efficacy, of course, is another critically important factor in stage-gate decisions. For PDPs and the products they are testing, efficacy is in essence context-dependent and deeply tied in with the everyday realities of their constituents: its calculation is reliant upon what drugs or vaccines are already out there, how high the prevalence rates and the burdens of suffering are, how many lives would be saved, and how soon something even better might make its way down the pipeline. As GSK's Voss put it, the criteria for what is efficacious cannot be written in stone. But he used GSK's malaria vaccine, RTS,S, at the time of our conversation in Phase III clinical trials, as an example of discussions that would be necessary for a tuberculosis vaccine. With RTS,S they have a roadmap that includes five-, ten-, and fifteen-year plans; at the time of our discussion the RTS,S vaccine was showing about 53 percent efficacy, but in fifteen years they hope to have a vaccine that is more like 80 percent effective. Why not just wait for the more effective vaccine, Voss asked. Because though 53 percent is not optimal, it still means saving potentially millions of people from a disease that affected an estimated 214 million people in 2015 (WHO 2016). For the TB as well as for the malaria vaccine, he added that the equation is variable across geographic regions: not only are results of clinical trials going to be slightly different in levels of efficacy, but interpretations of efficacy and the regulatory and policy decisions ensuing will vary according to disease burdens. The higher the burden, the lower the bar on what constitutes acceptable rates of efficacy (personal communication, July 6, 2012).

Indeed, his words were prescient. Since having that conversation, GSK's vaccine has finished its Phase III trial conducted across eleven African countries with 15,459 infant and child participants. The results were not even as optimistic as originally thought: efficacy was only 36 percent in the five- to seventeen-month-olds, and 26 percent in infants six to twelve weeks old (MVI 2015). And yet, a positive recommendation has come from the Committee for Medicinal Products for Human Use, the committee of the EMA that provides scientific opinions for medicines intended exclusively for markets outside the European Union but seeking EMA regulatory approval. In the final report, 1,774 cases of clinical malaria were prevented for every 1,000 vaccinated children over the forty-eight months of follow-up; and 983 cases out of every 1,000 vaccinated infants were prevented (MVI 2015).[7] The compelling numbers, rather than the less-compelling percentages, are what often drive decisions on approval of vaccines or drugs in countries where burdens of disease can be so high. In Aeras's 2014 Annual Report, Tom Evans echoes Voss in extolling the potential of the GSK tuberculosis vaccine for adolescents and adults. Having established the case that adolescents and adults are the primary transmitters of tuberculosis, Evans goes on to say that "even with an efficacy rate of just 60 percent with a 10-year duration of protection, M72/AS01E [the TB vaccine] delivered to just 20 percent of adults and adolescents globally could prevent approximately 50 million cases of TB in its first 25 years of use" (Aeras 2014).

Similar factors go into decisions concerning tuberculosis drug testing. States of scientific knowledge, levels of prevalence, rates of MDR-TB, and scaling-up capabilities all go into TB Alliance's campaign to produce drug combinations that will reduce treatment times for drug-susceptible tuberculosis from six to four months, and multidrug-resistant forms from two years to six months. There is little knowledge of how much of a difference two months will make in the ability to adhere to a drug regimen, nor is this kind of information easy to ascertain since a four-month regimen is unprecedented. What is known is that the first two months of the current regimen are the most difficult to adhere to, since more drugs are taken and more clinic visits are required than during the final four months (William Wells, former director of market access, TB Alliance, personal communication, April 25, 2012). Given this, a question similar to Voss's could understandably be raised: why not wait? The answer, like Voss's, is twofold: because people—lots of people—are dying in the meantime, and because this is just the initial step toward the end goal of getting TB drug regimens down to just two weeks (www.tballiance.org).

Getting closer to this goal is something the TB Drug Accelerator Program focuses on. Begun by the BMGF and partnering with several pharmaceutical companies, this initiative is boosting the number of tuberculosis compounds in the R&D pipeline for testing in combination. The end goal is to possibly reduce the number of drugs constituting a regimen from four to three, and to shorten substantially the duration of current treatments (Ken Duncan, deputy director, BMGF, personal communication, June 24, 2013). This and other initiatives such as the Open Lab outside of Madrid (and more on that below) are, however, focused on early discovery phases, and in the meantime there is a sense of urgency. Getting treatment down to four months, for now, thus still represents an achievement, however temporary, as assessed through potential numbers completing a regimen, number of MDR-TB cases thwarted through better adherence, and lower costs through a one-third reduction of time and pills taken.

Highlighting a very different facet of success, and one peculiar to Aeras and other tuberculosis vaccine researchers, McCown indirectly brought out the importance of geography for the vaccines manufactured at the Aeras plant. He mentioned that most vaccine batches are tested at higher temperatures: first in order to demonstrate stability at higher ambient temperatures such as their vaccines will likely encounter in destination countries; and second in a "forced degradation" evaluation (or accelerated stability) to get a better sense of a vaccine's stability profile sooner. Given the climates and infrastructures in many regions of heavy tuberculosis incidence, vaccines need to maintain stability under conditions of high ambient temperatures and unreliable refrigeration and freezing capacities. To this effect McCown showed me their lyophilizer, a machine that freeze-dries vaccine batches into cake form, which not only makes shipping logistically easier but extends expiration dates and precludes any need to freeze. Refrigeration is still required, but as he pointed out, consistent refrigeration is easier to achieve in low-income settings than freezing. In a subsequent room was a spray-dryer, making vaccine products into powder form, which has the advantage of providing a vaccine that can be administered by an inhaler rather than by syringe (personal communication, June 6, 2012). Indeed, the advantages of an aerosol vaccine in not needing refrigeration, better ease of transport, lower cost, and more efficient delivery are the multiple reasons why Aeras and others are currently prioritizing aerosol vaccines in tuberculosis research (www .aeras.org; Hanif and Garcia-Contreras 2012).

Temperature sensitivity in vaccines is not a new issue, as discussed in a recent WHO report on vaccine stability evaluation (2006b). However, with the exception of cold chain requirements—consistent refrigerated storage capacity for vaccines—standardized evaluation of vaccine stability and in particular of vaccine thermosensitivity remains lacking. The WHO's report thus aims for the first time to "provide the scientific basis and guiding principles" for evaluating the stability of vaccines for infectious diseases at multiple stages of development and production. Yet the authors are careful to state that their report remains a set of guidelines, not even recommendations, meaning that implementation in part or in whole of these guiding principles is up to the discretion of manufacturers. Perhaps because currently only about 18 percent of vaccines end up in countries within Africa, South America, and Asia (Kaddar 2010), that is, regions with high ambient temperatures and unpredictable electricity supplies, this report maintains that "stress testing of extreme environmental conditions" including temperature is not mandatory in vaccine stability evaluations. Instead, it leaves the issue with the anemic suggestion that such testing "should be considered" when a vaccine is intended for a market "where exposure to extreme temperature . . . is a real possibility" (WHO 2006b, 7). Accountability for Aeras, in this case as in many, has little to do with ICH requirements or other required metrics for regulatory approval. It has to do with accountability to the consumers whose lives they are aiming to improve. They thus follow the exigencies necessary to achieve this consistent bottom-line goal, including ensuring a vaccine that is viable and deliverable under real-life settings.

What becomes clear from these discussions is that success is a relative but also heavily symbolic concept within the larger PDP world of humanitarian desire, public health need, financial uncertainty, and immunological mysteries. Hinging as they do on so much more than clinical trial results or market predictions, "successful" tuberculosis drug regimens and vaccines possess overlapping but divergent informational and material environments than therapeutic candidates from the commercial pharmaceutical sector. In the political and philanthropic momentum giving form to these initiatives resides a judgment on the medical, financial, and political neglect that produced the conditions new therapeutics promise to amend. But beyond symbolism, numbers are the focus for calculations of success in the drugs and vaccines for a disease affecting so many millions. Here, the numerical metrics valued within philanthrocapitalism converge with the humanitarian goal of "making the biggest difference to the most people." If the molecular and biologic structures of new therapeutics contain the potential to keep millions of people alive, then they are successful not just as measured by BMGF, TB Alliance, and Aeras, but by regulatory agencies and scientific committees. As compelling as they might be, these numbers nevertheless are initial and promissory: they are stepping-stones to better vaccines and drugs that someday will be saving even more lives.

Returning to Barry's language, the environments PDP therapies encompass are considerably more expansive than commercial pharmaceuticals, extending beyond the material and legal to incorporate as well the symbolic and promissory. And within the material environment are expanded fields of logistical attention, recalibrations of success, and safety concerns. In all of these environments, vaccine and drug candidates become much more than potentially successful biotechnical interventions for tuberculosis; they become vehicles for long overdue infrastructural, institutional, and clinical redress.

The Scientific Value and Countervalue of Sharing

With the race to patent new discoveries before the competition does within mainstream pharmaceutical production comes a widespread unwillingness to share new knowledge. A greater degree of upstream patenting in recent years has meant even more and earlier protection of promising ideas, platforms, processes, and compounds. It is not surprising, then, that many scientists involved in tuberculosis PDPs extolled the more open culture characterizing tuberculosis research—that is, a culture distinguished by a willingness to share scientific insights, research results, challenges, and clinical successes. Sharing knowledge in the process of therapeutic research and development is a critical difference in humanitarian pharmaceutical production: within industry, knowledge contains the potential for money, and their strict proprietary practices are therefore about ensuring that knowledge remains as constrained in its travels as possible. With tuberculosis PDPs and their collaborators, the focus is not on *who* discovered new knowledge but on *what* the new discovery is and how it can be utilized in the goal of better therapies. Knowledge is a partial key or building block. It is partial because any particular new discovery or breakthrough is only a part of larger interconnecting realms of understanding; and a key because when leveraged with other partial knowledges it opens the way to new and potentially useful applications. Proprietary practices for PDPs like TB Alliance and Aeras thus enable controlled travel—that is, sharing knowledge among scientists, collaborations, and institutions that have the same agenda.

As noted by Dan Everitt, senior medical officer at TB Alliance, a major difference from his former job in industry was the openness with which those from pharmaceutical companies and even the FDA responded to him as an employee of TB Alliance. Unlike the very guarded way one pharmaceutical employee was likely to treat the questions of another industry employee, he could receive comprehensive and transparent answers to questions about particular practices or doing business in particular countries. Brainstorming could actually happen, as he suggested, because "there is a freedom [of communication] back and forth with not being part of a profit-centered company" (personal communication, July 15, 2013).

Similarly, David Barros-Aguirre, the easygoing head of GSK's DDW campus in Tres Cantos, Spain, spoke passionately of his unit's dedication to sharing knowledge. The point of the DDW campus is to focus on early-stage discovery of new drugs for tuberculosis, malaria, and kinetoplastid diseases (such as sleeping sickness) with financial expectations only that down the road, new therapeutics remain cost neutral. To this end, TB Alliance is a major funding partner, bankrolling a number of scientists full time for this early discovery-phase research. As Barros-Aguirre stressed, sharing new insights and early discoveries with other scientists at the facility and beyond is the norm at Tres Cantos. To create more opportunity for attracting new ideas and expertise to this mission of accelerated tuberculosis drug discovery, Wellcome Trust of the UK and GSK together funded a separate but integrated unit within Tres Cantos called the Open Lab Foundation, dedicated to bringing in scientists who have promising ideas and whose research would benefit from the resources at DDW.

The Open Lab exemplifies one variation of what Carl Nathan argues is an enormously promising model of pharmaceutical research: a model where academic researchers work from the earliest stages with industry scientists, combining the efficiencies and disciplinary expertise each possesses, and utilizing the greater resources of the pharmaceutical company. As Nathan put it, the earlier the team is broadened, the more efficient the process is, in part because what used to be done sequentially—one stage of the research process was completed, then handed over to the next scientist in a different department—is done simultaneously. And at the Open Lab anyone can come who meets the criteria, including people from biotech, government, and academia. They come inside the Open Lab in order to be able to "violate the usual rules of firewalls" in their scientific research (Nathan, personal communication, July 31, 2014).

These scientists, however, have to agree to the same approach to IP as is inscribed in the UN's World Intellectual Property Organization (WIPO) Re:Search Guidelines. These guidelines were constructed specifically to accelerate research on neglected diseases, tuberculosis, and malaria, and to ensure any new therapeutics or diagnostics for these diseases are made available to the populations who need them. IP within the guidelines, then, is designed to maximize rather than minimize circulation of medical knowledge and biotechnologies: participants agree to share research, patent discoveries as a way of maintaining their accessibility, and license the use of any products royalty free to others in the research and development community (www.wipo.int). Similarly, Barros-Aguirre stressed that at the DDW campus, they did not patent targets, enzymes, modes of action, or anything else upstream in the research and development process. As he put it, if you patent early, many other people will not get to know what you are doing, and you lose an opportunity for someone else to discover something that might make a real difference (personal communication, June 27, 2014). Patenting at the DDW campus only happens when they think they have a promising compound, after which the patent would be used to ensure low prices in low-income countries, and higher prices for European countries and the United States—a tiered pricing structure that enables collaborations such as the DDW and the Open Lab to make new drugs accessible in poorer countries, but continue funding their work in part through higher prices in wealthier countries. For the kinds of therapies they are developing, however, there will be very little market in higher-income countries. Unfortunately it was also clear that GSK has no control over what happens regarding proprietary practices once scientists have left the Open Lab or DDW programs; their hope is that these scientists and their institutions will stay true to the WIPO pledge of knowledge sharing, but outside the parameters of the Open Lab they have no way of ensuring that.

Across the nonprofit, international organization, and industry sectors, then, there is acknowledgment that scientific knowledge sharing is critical to acceleration of therapeutic discovery, thereby linking innovation with the absence of early and protectionist IP regimes: the WIPO Re:Search motto is "sharing innovation in the fight against neglected tropical diseases," while GSK's Open Lab website suggests that those working at DDW "share the belief in the need for an open-access, fresh-thinking and pragmatic approach . . . to creating medicines for diseases of the developed world" (www.openlabfoundation.org). The flip side of these proclamations is the tacit recognition that the fiercely protectionist IP practiced within the mainstream commercial pharmaceutical sector not only precludes development of therapies for nonlucrative diseases, but slows the research and development process itself by thwarting the circulation of scientific insights beneficial to discovery and development of new compounds and vaccines.

But the downsides don't stop there: protectionist IP also results in duplication of time, effort, and resources when scientists working within the commercial pharmaceutical sector are not aware of parallel research efforts at other companies, or when duplication is a purposeful approach within a company in order to speed the research process. Value is tied here with time as the interlocutor between a molecular compound and a profitable therapy. Embedded within the proprietary regimes of entities like the Open Lab, on the other hand, is the notion that molecular compounds and vaccine candidates hold the potential not only to save significant numbers of lives, but also to unlock knowledge potentially beneficial to other diseases and biotechnologies. Value thus is tied less to time and more to knowledge itself, with value increasing the further knowledge spreads across disciplinary and disease realms, and the more it leverages greater scientific understandings of pathogens in and outside of the human body. Martina Casenghi of MSF, along with Carl Nathan, has been trying to get more open-access initiatives like the Open Lab going within the PDP sector for several years. As she put it, in part it is so that academics researching tuberculosis can have access to those facets such as medicinal chemistry and chemical libraries that are helpful to proceeding with research, but that are typically unavailable to academics. In part it was also because even in the PDP world, IP practices can become more controlling further down the pipeline in order to keep products affordable (personal communication, July 30, 2009).

Unfortunately the increased potential for accelerated drug discovery provided by open-access workspaces and IP structures is not proving sufficiently attractive for the pharmaceutical industry outside of GSK. The original hope for the Open Lab Foundation was that other large pharmaceutical companies would leverage GSK monies by dedicating their own funds as well as scientists to the lab, thereby maximizing it as the engine of accelerated drug discovery that it was intended to be. Yet so far, no other company has shown interest. Though the reasons are no doubt varied, one hypothesis shared by Lluis Ballell, external opportunities director of DDW, is that to the extent that large pharmaceutical companies involve themselves in tuberculosis therapeutic research, they want the credit for doing so—that is, they want and need the social capital that comes with doing good. Because the Open Lab is both physically embedded in, and partially funded by, GSK, companies are concerned that they will be helping GSK get the credit for discoveries rather than accruing any for themselves (personal communication, June 17, 2014). Should this suggestion have merit, it signals some unfortunate but not surprising ironies of CSR as a motivator of tuberculosis research: that doing good primarily as a mode of acquiring social capital jeopardizes the good that can be done because it necessitates solitary R&D efforts. Solitary efforts, however, limit what can be accomplished both because scientific knowledge is not being shared and because resources are not being leveraged by other funders. The prohibitive expense of tuberculosis research then becomes an obstacle for further involvement or investment.

Even with a dedicated unit like the Tres Cantos DDW facility, then, investment remains a concern. This is true even though the emphasis within both the Open Lab and the DDW facility as a whole is early-stage drug discovery, stopping at Phase I trials testing for toxicological effects and optimal dosing. An early stage focus allows GSK to retain control over safety data important for eventual FDA or EMA approval should a candidate go that far, while avoiding the escalation of cost entailed in Phase II and III trials. The onus of cost neutrality even with early-stage research currently is eased by funding from the Wellcome Trust, the BMGF, European grants, and TB Alliance. And as of 2014, the EDCTP is expanding its parameters of funding. The EDCTP is a European–African partnership focused until recently on funding academic institutions and nonprofit organizations wanting to conduct clinical trials for tuberculosis (or malaria and HIV/AIDS) drug and vaccine candidates. Now, they are extending their grant donations to pharmaceutical companies, meaning that GSK's TB research stands a chance of acquiring another source of funding for clinical trials—in this case, later stage trials that would mean extending the research at DDW from lab to market.

Immune Logics

As Andrew Barry notes, in all pharmaceutical research there is by default a gap existing in how a molecular compound functions in the lab versus the human body. Again drawing from Bensaude-Vincent and Stengers (1996, 263), he underscores that chemical substances do not act in the "aseptic space of a laboratory" but in a "living labyrinth" that is the body embedded in intertwined and highly dynamic ecologies that have impact at the molecular and other levels (cited in Barry 2005, 57). As scientists across a number of fields are becoming ever more attuned to, everything from air quality, food, soil constitution, education, health care, discrimination, and work-related stress have impacts in various ways on the body. Genetic makeup, metabolism, and immune system functioning are all shaped by these many and interacting environmental factors. But in addition, intelligibility of the "living labyrinth" that includes clinical trials and their human participants is complicated in the case of tuberculosis by a number of factors. More discussion of clinical trials follows in the next chapter. Here, after some explanation of what makes tuberculosis trials particularly tricky, I restrict my discussion of trials to the challenges they pose at the level of the immune system.

Because current tuberculosis drugs are 95 percent effective when administered properly, it is difficult to statistically prove the efficacy of a new compound against drug-susceptible strains of the bacillus without enrolling huge numbers of individuals to procure data that is statistically significant. Current knowledge of *M. tuberculosis* also falls short of fully understanding which among an array of immune responses actually protects the human body against infection with the bacterium and the onset of disease. Related to this point, there is the problem of having no biomarker to use in clinical trials: lower bacteria counts in sputum, while presumably a logical metric of success in a drug candidate, have proven over time to be untrustworthy (Nunn 2010; Diacon, personal communication, March 25, 2011). Early-stage drug trials do currently depend on bactericidal activity (i.e., ability of drugs to kill the TB bacterium) shown in a two-week time span even though researchers agree that this is not particularly predictive of efficacy in later stages (Barros-Aguirre, personal communication, June 27, 2014; Jan Gheuens, deputy director of TB drugs at BMGF, personal communication, June 24, 2013; Diacon, personal communication, March 25, 2011). For late-stage trials, researchers typically are forced to use endpoints, or agreed-upon clinical indicators of efficacy, that can be unsatisfactory on clinical, financial, and humanitarian levels. The endpoint typically is to track how many trial participants eventually die of the disease, which in turn requires a two-year follow-up. Agencies thus are realizing the need to focus more funding on research into basic immunological and pathophysiological facets of *M. tuberculosis*, with the FDA and the BMGF both awarding significant grants in recent years to better elucidate what constitutes effective immune responses to the tuberculosis bacterium and to find a reliable biomarker.

M. tuberculosis also complicates intelligibility because of the variable way it behaves across geographies. Rates of primary infection in India, for example, are 62 percent while in South Africa they are only 19 percent.[8] China's highest tuberculosis burden is among fifty- to sixty-year-olds rather than the younger constituencies in other countries; and South Africa has the highest rates of tuberculosis coinfection with HIV (Evans 2011). With recent advances in mycobacterial genomics and population genetics, together with tools enabling high-resolution genotyping of the bacterium, there is also increased awareness that *M. tuberculosis* has different strains that are variously distributed geographically (Gagneux and Small 2007). It has led to the recognition that populations, including across high-burden regions within Asia, Africa, and South America, respond differently to the tuberculosis bacterium itself, as well as to drug and vaccine candidates being tested (Barros-Aguirre, personal communication, June 27, 2014).

The inadequate knowledge of what protective immune responses look like was made clearer during my tours of various laboratories involved in the analysis of blood samples from tuberculosis vaccine and drug trials. During my tour of the Aeras facility, Andrew Graves, a research specialist in immunology, showed me how blood samples were analyzed. After receiving specimens carefully labeled as to which field site and what day blood was collected, scientists stimulate them with antigens found in the experimental vaccines. They then stain the cells after six hours, with fluorescently labeled antibodies against specific biomarkers. The cells are run through a machine called a flow cytometer, which effectively categorizes the samples by cell type and what cytokines (immune signals) they are giving off; this data is then sent to computer monitors. To get baselines for comparison, they have a negative control sample that is unstimulated (i.e., no immune response) as well as a positive control (i.e., full response). The machine Aeras possesses has a capacity to detect up to eighteen colors, meaning that it can read up to eighteen different immune responses or biomarkers.[9] The assay performed at Aeras examines thirteen markers (Graves, personal communication, June 6, 2012).

The markers they look at include CD4 helper T cells and CD8 cytotoxic T cells, both thought to be important in protection against tuberculosis. The monitor showed the percentage of these various cells that responded to the antigens. Yet as I looked at the colored lines on the computer screen, Graves admitted that what they can tell from this data is exactly what the immune response was in reaction to various tuberculosis antigens; at this stage, however, they cannot know which if any of these responses actually confer protection. The hope is that with the volume of data being generated during these trials, biostatisticians will be able, finally, to find a correlate of protection: that is, they will discern which exact immune responses are the ones that confer immune protection against *M. tuberculosis*. In the meantime, scientists analyze blood samples from those participants across trial sites who displayed reduced infection or disease rates in order to begin piecing together the commonalities among them in immune response. At the time I was touring the Aeras facility, blood samples from six different vaccine trials were being analyzed (Graves, personal communication, June 6, 2012).

At the high throughput screening facility at the DDW campus outside of Madrid, Julio Martin, the director of screening and compound profiling, showed me computer monitors displaying similar colored graphs of the responses of *M. tuberculosis* to compounds from the GSK compound library. Like the Aeras lab, there are controls to compare results against: a compound against which the bacterium has no response, and a compound that has a robust response against the bacterium. The colors on the screen each represent the percent of bactericidal activity of a particular compound, measured against the two controls. Martin had just walked me through what they call the factory, a completely automated laboratory where a robotic arm brings particular compounds in liquid suspension from the chemical library (holding facility), and these compounds are then precisely squirted into the tiny wells of a plate. Those plates are then transferred to another enclosed and sealed area where the biologic—in this case, tuberculosis bacteria—is squirted into each of the same wells where the compounds have just been placed. The plates are incubated for the period of time it takes the bacteria to replicate, after which they are counted, and the results are sent to the database and displayed on the monitors. Scientists then read across the compounds to see if there are similarities in chemical structure among those displaying good bactericidal activity, and if so, how these can subsequently be optimized, such as by improving solubility, stability, etc. To make sure scientists are getting the most promising compounds, Martin asserted that their preference was to have all 1.8 million compounds in the GSK DDW library screened (personal communication, June 17, 2014).

And finally, scientists are conducting multiple immunological studies with varying approaches at SATVI in Cape Town. Cheryl Day, a senior research officer at SATVI, described her research analyzing blood samples from at least four different tuberculosis vaccine trials ongoing at the time at SATVI—the Aeras 404 and 402, MVA85A, and GSK's M72. Like at Aeras, blood samples are first stimulated with various antigens and then analyzed as to the immune responses that can be read. They also look at cytokine response among others, but Day confirmed what Graves indicated—that with tuberculosis the dearth of knowledge about immune responses means a very iterative process where efficacy data from each vaccine trial is mined to pick apart the exact immune responses to each vaccine in order to then be better informed in reading the data coming from each blood sample. Then scientists in that way eventually can begin figuring out the logic of protective immune responses (Day, personal communication, March 23, 2011).

The Regime of Regimens

In the meantime, research continues, as do innovations in other areas including a tactic to save time and money: testing regimens instead of single drugs. TB Alliance has been at the forefront of developing this new model of drug testing, understandably touting what they call their New Combination or NC trials where drug regimens rather than single drugs are tested. As mentioned in the previous chapter, TB Alliance has begun testing one combination of drugs—PA-824, pyrazinamide, and bedaquiline—in a Phase IIb trial, but they are testing another regimen as well: PA-824, moxifloxacin, and pyrazinamide. Not only does testing drugs as regimens more accurately reflect the reality of treating tuberculosis, it also shaves years off of clinical trial times because single new drugs are not tested sequentially. These innovations, however, also come with their own set of challenges involving the need for more compounds, resources, and industry involvement. The Critical Path to TB Drug Regimens (CPTR) was begun to try and address some of those challenges.

CPTR is a consortium launched in 2010 by the BMGF, the Critical Path Institute (a nonprofit organization created by the University of Arizona and the FDA), and TB Alliance to expedite testing and development of new tuberculosis drug regimens all the way through late-stage trials. As observed by Jan Gheuens, deputy director of TB drugs at BMGF and primary driving force in creating the consortium, CPTR's structure was designed to encompass all relevant players including industry and regulatory agencies given that pharmaceutical companies would be critical to regimen development because of their huge compound libraries and expertise. Regulatory agencies, in turn, would be key to the eventual rollout of successful new regimens. The Critical Path Institute already had experience in bringing varied partners together for other diseases, so their experience was tapped for tuberculosis R&D. CPTR now encompasses four pillars: regulatory, drug development, diagnostics, and research resources.

Like Aeras and TB Alliance, CPTR is involved in de-risking: they are attempting to make participation in the consortium more appealing to industry at the same time that they are advancing critical areas of tuberculosis research. After the recent spate of pharmaceutical divestment in tuberculosis, CPTR members spoke with industry R&D heads about what would entice them to stay invested. As stated by Debra Hanna, executive director of CPTR, they heard "loud and clear" that companies wanted better tools to determine the combinations of compounds most likely to succeed in clinical trials and receive FDA approval (personal communication, July 16, 2014). Hence, the regulatory arm of CPTR is focusing on redesigning clinical trials to be smaller in size, shorter in duration, and more predictive of success at later stages. The result would be trials that are less costly in both time and money, but more convincing investments since drug candidates would have greater chance of success than currently holds true.

The starting point is getting partners to pool clinical trial data that can inform new tools such as clinical trial simulations and lung models. Once again, IP frameworks are key: like the Open Lab, CPTR has developed over the last four years an IP structure that allows industry to share their data in a "safe way" with other partners in the consortium, with little risk that it will leak to outside members of the pharmaceutical industry or scientific community. The IP requirements at CPTR in effect allow pharmaceutical companies to play both sides: to be actors in the nonprofit world of tuberculosis drug regimen development on the one hand, and market-driven companies pursuing highly protective proprietary regimes for lucrative discoveries on the other. The insights gleaned from this pooled data in turn inform the design of tools that essentially take some of drug testing out of human bodies and into computers. As Hanna indicated, companies have been developing these tools for use in other diseases, but have had no incentive until now to develop them for tuberculosis.

Clinical trial simulations, for example, allow scientists to better determine the effect of dosing schedules on trial designs by running "thousands of variables without being in human bodies" (Hanna, personal communication, July 16, 2014). A hollow fiber tool is being designed for preclinical stages to more accurately inform which chemical entities to test in regimens and to better determine dose selection. Lung models will help elucidate drug penetration into all areas of the lungs including those areas where nonreplicating tuberculosis bacteria hide; they will also show how new mechanisms of action work. Another tool being developed is a population/pharmacokinetics model to address variable drug metabolization across populations: the model is intended to help determine those metabolism components likely to be most prevalent in high-burden countries. Simulating how humans metabolize tuberculosis drugs is an intended improvement on, and circumvention of, animal models that fulfill standard regulatory requirements of preclinical safety and efficacy testing, but that in the case of tuberculosis do not always accurately predict drug metabolism or efficacy in humans. As of 2016, some of these nonclinical drug development tools, as they are called, are getting regulatory approval (CPTR 2016). Like GSK's DDW and the Open Lab, all tools and any other research resulting from work done within

CPTR is required to be open and accessible to the broader scientific community (CPTR 2016), once again recognizing both the enhanced innovatory potential of sharing scientific knowledge and the humanitarian goal of broadly deploying the products of that knowledge.

The FDA's support of regimen approval is a key step for all the partners involved in CPTR. Since the advent of ARV drug regimens for people living with AIDS, the FDA has been urged to rethink its drug approval process. A report to the FDA's Science Board in 2007 declared that the agency's practice of approving single drugs had not kept pace with the reality that many diseases, including cancer, AIDS, and tuberculosis, required regimens. By the launch of CPTR, the FDA's commissioner, Margaret Hamburg, proclaimed her support of drug regimen approval, conceding that this change in policy was part of a bigger issue of strengthening regulatory science to keep pace with advances in research and development (CPTR 2010a). Testing and getting new drugs approved as regimens rather than one drug at a time reduces the time to market by at least a third, not an insignificant improvement given trial and approval times. There are downsides to the new model, however, namely that it can be difficult when testing multiple drugs at the same time to know which drug is responsible if side effects occur, to know with certainty which drugs would make the most effective combination given current reliance on two-week initial stage trials, or to have flexibility in altering regimens in individual cases of failure (Barros-Aguirre, personal communication, June 27, 2014; Ballell, personal communication, June 17, 2014).

Structurally, CPTR gains potentially critical advantage by enabling cross-institutional research that can equal more than the sum of its parts. TB Alliance previous to the CPTR agreement, for example, could forge only bilateral agreements with its industry partners, something they continue to do but to which they are now not limited. With CPTR, these agreements extend to multilateral relations where pharmaceutical partners are not just sharing compounds with TB Alliance but with each other, with or without TB Alliance collaboration. CPTR thus answers to some extent the contention of Martina Casenghi that despite the promise offered by PDPs, there remain too many barriers to the open scientific communications necessary across players if new initiatives in tuberculosis therapeutic development are going to prove successful (Casenghi, personal communication, July 30, 2009). Finally, the CPTR opens the way for manufacturing fixed-dose combination (FDC) pills formed by compounds developed jointly within the consortium or donated by responsible pharmaceutical companies. FDCs, as their name suggests, combine all the drugs of an effective regimen into one tablet, thereby simplifying regimens by reducing the number of pills needing to be ingested. Simplifying regimens is one key to better adherence and less drug resistance in tuberculosis, and CPTR represents a better mechanism for gaining FDC capability than the alternative—bilateral agreements between TB Alliance and multiple pharmaceutical companies (Gardiner, personal communication, November 29, 2011).

With unfortunate irony, advances in science have also offered pharmaceutical companies a way to remain involved in tuberculosis research for the sake of appearing socially responsible, but without necessarily investing expertise, finances, or effort. As Bronwyn Parry describes in her book *Trading the Genome,* in the mid-1990s a method combining computer software, chemistry, and automated technology was employed to create thousands of new compounds. Starting with promising elements, computers could put together the basic structures and information of these elements to create compounds that not only are patentable since they are engineered but would be more promising in terms of efficacy. Assays in turn were created to test the potency, tissue penetration, absorption, and other facets of these new compounds (Parry 2004). Those compounds that prove promising against intended targets are pursued as candidates for the commercially viable development pipeline. The rest end up in compound libraries such as the one mentioned above at GSK's DDW facility, filled with hundreds of thousands if not millions of compounds incorporating within their molecular structures the possibility of combating diseases outside of commercial interest. Possession of these compounds gives companies the opportunity to open their libraries to other researchers in a substantive way that includes providing analytical expertise and laboratory facilities along with the compounds; or alternatively, making libraries available to researchers, including those searching for tuberculosis drug candidates, with little else in the way of support. As researchers at DDW suggested, the current political climate for the pharmaceutical sector is such that "what you cannot be is outside [of infectious disease initiatives]," but compound libraries make it possible for some companies to commit to initiatives like CPTR that gain them social capital with minimal engagement (Barros-Aguirre, personal communication, June 27, 2014; Ballell, personal communication, June 17, 2014).

The disinvestment of industry from tuberculosis research, along with the opportunity to do good while doing very little, both play roles in creating a paucity of new drug compounds available to produce a regimen. A drug regimen constituted by all new drugs each with new mechanisms of action is what Barros-Aguirre and Ballell argue is necessary for intervening in both drug-susceptible and multidrug-resistant forms of tuberculosis, and in all high-burden regions with their diverse patterns of drug susceptibility and resistance (Ballell, personal communication, June 17, 2014). GSK has a candidate coming into Phase I trials, but they will not want to advance it further down the pipeline if there are not enough other viable candidates to produce a regimen. Currently, there is only Janssen's new patented bedaquiline, TB Alliance's PA-824, and Otsuka's delamanid. Yet for unclear reasons Otsuka does not intend to collaborate with PDPs or other pharmaceutical companies, perhaps because its compound uses the same mechanism of action as PA-824, meaning that the two drugs are in direct competition. More to the point here, it also means they are not suitable for the same regimen.

This dearth of new candidates almost certainly plays a role in why TB Alliance is moving into Phase III clinical trials a regimen containing only one new drug, their PA-824, along with pyrazinamide and moxifloxacin (PaMZ). The combination so far has shown promise in treating all forms of tuberculosis while reducing treatment times. Yet it is likely to have limited marketability in two high-burden regions, Russia and much of Asia including India, because these areas have high rates of resistance to fluoroquinolones—a category of antibacterial drug that includes moxifloxacin. The Treatment Action Group (TAG) 2014 Pipeline Report raises this criticism, arguing that 38 to 53 percent of people with MDR-TB are resistant to pyrazinamide, yet TB Alliance is including an MDR-TB arm in their trials of the PA-824, moxifloxacin, pyrazinamide regimen (Clayden et al. 2014). Mark Harrington, executive director of TAG, elaborates: if individuals are resistant to isoniazid and rifampicin, which is the definition of MDR-TB, they are likely to be resistant to pyrazinamide as well. So, those individuals in the MDR arm of this Phase III trial are likely to be getting only two drugs that work, and this is undertreating these patients. TB Alliance and BMGF are working on a rapid test for determining pyrazinamide resistance, but right now they do not have one. So, there is no equipoise for this trial—that is, the MDR arm is not getting the same standard of treatment as the other arms (Harrington, personal communication, November 20, 2014). TB Alliance also carried out a Phase III trial called REMox, testing moxifloxacin in combination with three other first-line TB drugs with no new drug candidate. The purpose was to see if adding moxifloxacin would reduce treatment times from six to four months in drug-sensitive tuberculosis patients. Though the enhanced regimen did show quicker reductions in mycobacterium, it ultimately failed to reduce treatment times as evidenced in relapse rates (www.tballiance.org).

Like the discussion above about the complex contours of what defines success in tuberculosis research, TB Alliance's decision reflects current realities of where research is and will likely be in the future. Stephen Gillespie, principle investigator in the REMox trial, noted in response to the objection concerning large geographical swathes of resistance that TB Alliance is working in the meantime to enhance and expedite the drug compound pipeline. As such, he noted while the trial was still ongoing that "it might be a short to medium term for REMox in terms of life expectancy for a treatment, but it is also creating the methodologies and techniques to have something to take its place. It is a continuum, in this arms race with the bacteria" (personal communication, July 30, 2013). Once again, a therapy able to save lives even in one geographically delimited set of high-burden countries and for a delimited period buys time for newer and hopefully more effective regimens to be developed—assuming that the necessary "material and legal environments" coalesce.

Conclusion

The moral economy of access, as Peter Redfield describes the situation of insufficient drugs to combat "unprofitable conditions," incorporates a productive tension between a humanitarian ideal that "lives should not depend on the price or availability of medication," and the fact that producing and disseminating those medications requires "attention to an expanding universe of detail" (2013, 203). Pursuing therapeutic production for TB Alliance, Aeras, CPTR, and the Tres Cantos DDW and Open Lab exemplifies such an expansion of a universe of detail. They expand scientific and social value of vaccine candidates and drug compounds, for example, by incorporating open access IP, sharing knowledge and expertise, forging regulatory changes, and targeting public health need in research and development directives. Disruptive innovation does indeed happen when researchers are able to work together inside of environments that stimulate scientific cross-fertilization, creativity, and recalibrations of time, and that allow for failure because the end goal is getting the best products for the lowest cost to the most people rather than something like the opposite.

Thus the rich legal and economic information contained within the molecules of new tuberculosis therapeutics, to use Barry's framework, distinguishes them in critically important ways from their commercial pharmaceutical counterparts. Drug and vaccine candidates possess within those environments a great deal of social, political, and promissory capital. But they also contain hope, and the passion imbued by scientists, some of whom have sacrificed more lucrative careers to dedicate themselves to unraveling the mysteries of *M. tuberculosis* or to get the next vaccine candidate right. And research on the immune system, along with information from clinical trials, is providing clues into the molecular impacts of poverty—a discovery going well beyond a single disease to raise questions like how chronic undernutrition might impinge on drug metabolism or why some forms of deprivation negatively impact immune systems more than other forms. The collaborations behind tuberculosis therapies that reach across disciplines and institutions go well beyond tuberculosis research as well, providing vital pathogenic, genetic, and immune system information useful in any number of infectious and other diseases.

So far, the innovative potential inhering in the collaborations described in this chapter are evidenced primarily within the scientific domains of early discovery—namely, the increasing numbers of compounds and vaccine candidates in preclinical stages, increased understandings of immune system response and effect, and computer simulations and modeling systems to improve predictive capacities of promising drug regimens, vaccine candidates, and early-stage testing. The reason, in part, for this bulge at the beginning of the pipeline is the relative newness of especially CPTR and the Open Lab. Yet new knowledge is being generated down the pipeline as well, if at a somewhat slower pace. Even when trials fail in their intended goals, the data they generate can be enormously helpful in a scientific process that is highly iterative. The immune responses from blood samples read by Andrew Graves and his team at Aeras, and Cheryl Day and others at SATVI, will ultimately reveal much about which immune responses are key in fighting the tuberculosis bacterium and which are not. This understanding then shapes the next round of candidates for trials. In the same iterative process, biomarkers will eventually be found and indeed have tentatively already been found (Fletcher et al. 2016) for indicating success or failure earlier in clinical trials. The two advances of immune and biomarker research together will result in diminished expense of moving therapies down the pipeline, while also ensuring that therapies are better designed to succeed.

The precariousness that to some degree limits the potential of humanitarian pharmaceutical production will remain an issue as long as funding for late-stage candidates remains unstable—a point made in the previous chapter as well. The continued hesitance of industry to be more engaged in tuberculosis research, and their enhanced ability to perform very rudimentary CSR rather than engage in truly socially responsible efforts, is having its effect at all stages of research. This comes at a time when TB Alliance in particular is increasing its clinical trials to respond to recent calls for attention to pediatric treatment (www.tballiance.org). There is an understandable reluctance to include children in pharmaceutical testing, but the result of that reluctance is the absence of drugs that are specifically tested for efficacy and appropriate dosing in this population. This is despite the fact that children constitute a sizeable percentage of tuberculosis cases globally, and an estimated four hundred thousand cases of MDR-TB infection (McKenna 2015). As clinicians know, it is not just about cutting the doses down: children metabolize pharmaceuticals differently, and the need to include them in clinical trials is overpowering the understandable impulse not to. Accordingly, several trials are now underway or planned to include infants, children, and adolescents—HIV positive and negative—in clinical trials for existing front-line drugs, new drugs, and preventive regimens (McKenna 2015).

Tuberculosis PDPs are trying hard to counteract the contradictions within the moral economy of access, and the research on immune systems and innovative collaborations highlighted in this chapter are going some distance in paving the way to diminishing expenses of research. Focusing on vaccines that prevent infection instead of disease, as has heretofore been the focus, is another example since this allows shorter and smaller trials because it is possible to detect new cases of tuberculosis quickly and reliably (www.aeras.org). The totality of financial, partner, collaborative, and scientific innovations described in this and the previous chapter have meant the decided progress of humanitarian pharmaceutical production, just not at an optimal pace. But time, when counted in lives lost, can create tensions over whether to focus on basic research on immune systems and biomarkers, or advanced-stage clinical trials. This is a telling tension only characterizing unprofitable diseases that have long existed outside the remit of science: that is, is it better to save some lives now, however imperfectly, or more lives later with better designed therapies?

3 THE CONTINGENT ETHICS OF TUBERCULOSIS CLINICAL TRIALS

IN 2012 I TRAVELED TO CAPE TOWN to visit SATVI, a University of Cape Town–based organization specializing in conducting clinical trials, including vaccine trials sponsored by Aeras. I was there to learn more about how SATVI and Aeras designed and conducted their trials—how they recruited participants, trained staff, and worked with the community. At the time I was there, the Phase IIb trial for the tuberculosis vaccine candidate MVA85A was underway, having successfully enrolled 2,800 infants.

Clinical trials play key roles in new pharmaceutical research and development, whether commercial or noncommercial. Yet they are also inherently controversial given the risks to human participants in biomedical research and the inequitable institutional and economic contexts in which trials are increasingly conducted. Commercial clinical trials have come under greater scrutiny recently in a surge of scholarship investigating pharmaceutical practices of outsourcing trials to Eastern Europe, South America, Asia, or Africa. In these regions, it is understood, pharmaceutical companies are likely to find large populations of poor individuals with little access to other drugs, inadequate health care, and higher rates of particular diseases (Petryna 2009; Sunder Rajan 2006; Fisher 2008; Glickman et al. 2009), which in turn means better data not muddied by drug–drug interactions and more likelihood of enrolling in clinical trials as a means to access health care.[1] Communities participating in these clinical trials are rarely the intended consumers, leading to ethical questions about the use of poor populations in medical research they will not benefit from (Petryna 2009).

Tuberculosis clinical trials obviously are not commercially sponsored, but they share the fact that they are located in impoverished regions even though this is because poverty is key to producing relevant knowledge since one of its major outcomes is tuberculosis. Within this context, I wanted to better evaluate what these trials were doing differently scientifically and ethically. In addition to the innovations involving drug regimens, were there other innovations happening in the design of tuberculosis clinical trials? Were standard aspects of trial protocol such as informed consent approached differently? Were communities involved in the process other than as potential participants? Were they, in other words, responding to recent scholarship on noncommercial clinical trials that raises questions about the nature and impact of scientific research on participating communities? Many scholars have begun to ask how these trials might go beyond standard medical guidelines that dictate doing no harm, to actually benefiting communities beyond the therapy being tested. In her article "Taking as Giving" (2007), for example, Cori Hayden suggests that in the highly unequal nature of clinical research and its close associations with abusive colonial medical histories, clinical trials can too easily be about extracting knowledge with little regard for sharing the benefits of this knowledge, much less giving back to research communities. For years, in fact, the prevailing assumption within research circles has been that individuals participate in clinical trials out of altruism, a move that deftly erases the uneven power and political relations inhering in experimental structures. With greater awareness and increasing visibility of its exploitative nature comes more thought on what it means not just to include participants in clinical trials, but to include them *well*, a concept Hayden takes from the anthropologist Marilyn Strathern (2000, cited in Hayden 2007, 733). What would it mean to think about trials where participants had more voice, or where benefits accrued not just to the researchers but to participants and their communities? How to define what benefits mean in different communities, how they would be distributed, over what period of time, and who would be responsible are subsequent questions needing evaluation (Engel et al. 2014; Lairumbi et al. 2008; Hayden 2007).

Informed consent has also come under increasing scrutiny for how appropriate its current format is in different settings, as well as how effective it is as an arbiter of biomedical integrity and human subject protection. Institutional review boards continue to follow the lead of the major medical ethics guidelines on informed consent such as the Nuremberg Code or the Helsinki Declaration even though these documents do not question the preeminence of the individual or take into consideration broader social and economic circumstances conditioning processes of consent (Akrong, Horstman, and Arhinful 2014; Gikonyo et al. 2008; Sariola and Simpson 2011). Scholars again are bringing needed awareness to the fact that even in trials that are testing therapies intended for the communities participating in research, the conditions and relations of inequality, the geopolitics of Western-sponsored research conducted in low-income regions, and the political economies of deprivation qualifying communities for clinical trials in the first place set the stage for exploitation. Within these contexts, the very meaning and practice of "informed" and "consent" are indelibly shaped by levels of education, access to resources, and patterns of enfranchisement.

What I found in my conversations with researchers and staff in Worcester, and in subsequent conversations with members of TB Alliance and others involved in tuberculosis trials, is that these organizations go some distance in moving beyond do not harm in their approaches to accountability, purpose, and impact in conducting clinical trials. They approach potential participants not as objects of scientific and marketing expediency, but as communities with voices, demands, and questions to be answered about trial design and purpose as contingencies of participation. This in turn drives endeavors such as creating community advisory boards (CABs) to relay concerns between researchers and trial communities, and deliberating an informed consent document that takes seriously what "informed" and "consent" mean in the context of low-resource, high-morbidity settings. They also engage communities before and during trials through educational outreach and awareness raising, clinic and laboratory enhancements, staff training, and other forms of capacity building.

But I also eventually recognized that TB Alliance, Aeras, and SATVI operate within a larger milieu of regulatory, institutional, and scientific requirements placing limits on what is possible in rethinking the design and conduct of clinical trials within a humanitarian pharmaceutical model. Standardized guidelines for conducting clinical trials, for example, limit the degree of innovation possible when testing new pharmaceuticals that must ultimately gain FDA and EMA approval. Requirements of harmonization and standardization of data across geographically diverse trial sites answer very valid concerns about scientific integrity, consumer protection, and marketability. Yet answering to these concerns in turn can downplay the peculiarities of place and people involved in clinical trials, including geographical variations in pathogen subtypes, comorbidities, varying nutritional levels, drug metabolism, and the particular contours of everyday precariousness in poor communities. Other requirements such as publication notification rules and sponsor specifications also contour aspects of trials in ways that are not always beneficial to participants or local scientists.

As I highlight various practices and procedures of tuberculosis clinical trials in elaborating on the argument above, I also respond to the critique that clinical trial sites create enclaves of medical care within broader landscapes of deprivation (Sparke 2014) and emphasize technologies rather than broader social and economic interventions. Aeras and TB Alliance do not presume to be initiating broad-scale economic or social interventions, nor do they generate explicit rhetoric about biotechnologies singlehandedly solving problems of entrenched poverty. Nevertheless, the agglomerative effects of their approach to clinical trial location and development, participant recruitment, and trial conduct make it more difficult to maintain stark dichotomies between enclave versus dispersed impact and technological versus socioeconomic emphasis.

Finally, I address a conundrum particular to tuberculosis and other neglected disease research within current global health initiatives. That is, what happens when new infusions of money for pharmaceutical research confront decades of research neglect? In the last chapter, I discussed this around determining success in trials of new therapies through (high) numbers saved rather than (relatively low) percentages. Here, I argue that this confrontation raises new ethical questions about the balance between basic science and clinical trials when so little is known about the bacterium. How might going ahead with trials when knowledge of *M. tuberculosis* is still inadequate threaten not just the success of trials but also hope, promise, and community attitudes?

Before elaborating on these arguments, a point of clarification is necessary. Namely, contestations over the form and role of clinical trials are certainly not new. In fact clinical trials for many reasons have consistently been sites of controversy, which in turn have at times led to changes in clinical trial design. As Harry Marks noted in his landmark history of clinical trials in the United States (1997), the first randomized, controlled trial (RCT) was actually conducted in the United States in the 1940s, ironically to test the merits of streptomycin against tuberculosis. Previous to this, groups of individuals were typically given a new therapy, and physicians would observe the response. RCTs' innovation was to randomly assign a prescribed number of participants to either a control group taking the established therapy or a placebo and the experimental group tak-ing the therapy being tested. Yet as Marks noted, this new form of clinical research heavily influenced by the rise of statistics was not immediately accepted by all of the medical community. Eventually, however, research-ers recognized the benefits of randomization and the role of statistical significance in eliminating individual bias from therapeutic evaluation. By the end of the 1950s, the RCT was largely acknowledged as the best instrument for producing objective scientific evidence of therapeutic efficacy. The FDA in turn underscored this role by adopting RCTs as the standard of proof for evaluating new drugs and vaccines for regulatory approval. It is still the accepted gold standard of biomedical research.

As Marks points out, institutionalizing RCTs as the scientific standard for medical experimentation meant overlooking the statistical nuances originally characterizing RCT analysis. It also meant eliding valid contes-tations against RCT design, such as when physicians protested the exis-tence of control arms when they simply wanted the best therapy for their patients (Marks 1997). Despite the heightened objectivity afforded by RCTs and their reliance on statistical significance, Marks insightfully notes that "there remains a gap between the world of methodological dicta and the social realities of clinical research." And as such, "even the simplest RCT is the product of a negotiated social order, replete with decisions—some contested, some not—and with unexamined assump-tions" (1997, 134). More recent emphasis on standardization and harmo-nization of late-stage clinical trials across multiple sites multiplies the tension between rigidly standardized trial designs and the many particu-larities of social politics and practice inhering in different localities. As I describe in this chapter, including patients well is itself a negotiated social order that is limited by, and in tension with, scientific and regula-tory requirements, the contradictory necessities of poverty, and institu-tional and organizational contingencies of trial protocol. One of the things I attempt to do in this chapter is to highlight some of the assump-tions that either remain relatively unexamined in PDP clinical trials or that have been scrutinized but have not yet found a productive resolution.

The ongoing contestation over how trials should be designed and conducted—the social order they should assume—plays a significant role in a humanitarian pharmaceutical production model. It is not enough to develop new drugs and vaccines that might ease the suffering of millions with tuberculosis; if these new therapies were tested under conditions less than ethical to trial participants, then this would be a major flaw in the model. Later-phase trials in particular enroll tens of thousands of individuals from chronically resource-deprived regions, making the question of including participants well an even more trenchant one.

Aside from the MVA85A trial, there are a few others to point out that either recently completed or are set to begin. The comments and questions I raise about the failed vaccine trial hold for these as well. Most noteworthy of TB Alliance's trials includes the Phase III REMox trial mentioned in the previous chapter. Though substituting moxifloxacin for one of the main first-line drugs (i.e., isoniazid or rifampicin) ultimately failed to shorten treatment by the expected two months, TB Alliance maintains that the trial was nevertheless a success in other ways. For one thing, it succeeded in establishing robust trial sites across nine countries that meet GCP standards—a level of trial standardization across sites required for FDA and EMA regulatory approval of any new therapy. It also netted a biobank of blood specimens providing further material for finding new biomarkers, as well as other data that can deepen understanding of which factors are predictive of the outcomes of clinical trials (www.tballiance .org). This kind of information mining in the aftermath of failed trials— that is, using the data and blood samples collected to further understandings of immune protection and bacterial behaviors—characterizes other trials as well, such as the MVA85A trial. In this regard, failure again plays a positive role. Pinpointing those immune responses to a drug or vaccine candidate that did not prove protective is just as useful as analyzing immune responses to therapies that did.

Though currently on clinical hold in part from inadequate funding, the pending Phase III trial testing pyrazinamide, moxifloxacin, and TB Alliance's PA-824 or pretomanid (PaMZ) is highly ambitious, covering a planned fifty sites across Africa, Asia, Eastern Europe, and Central and South America. The hopes for this combination are high: that it will reduce treatment times for both drug-susceptible and some forms of MDR-TB to four months, harmonize regimens for both forms of tuberculosis to an FDC of three pills, eliminate the need for painful injections in the case of MDR-TB, and provide a better treatment option to TB patients who are also on ARVs (www.tballiance.org). The trial was halted over safety issues, but recently the independent Safety Monitoring Board has recommended that the trial resume (Thomas Lynch, communications manager, TB Alliance, personal communication, August 1, 2016). As a side note, the fact that TB Alliance does not reveal on its website why the PaMZ trial is on hold points to the multiple roles tuberculosis PDP websites play. They certainly serve to inform a broad set of constituencies on who they are and what they are doing, including the partnerships they forge and the research they perform. But in conveying this information they consistently forefront the positive: the many collaborations, the breakthroughs, the optimism of new research. In a landscape of inadequate funding and unknowing publics, information cannot just educate, it has to galvanize potential donors. Suspended or failed trials, however scientifically productive, do not convey the successes and promises that business-model philanthropies and industries need to see to rationalize their investments.

Getting back to clinical trials, Aeras currently has no Phase III trial planned for a vaccine candidate, but there are a number of candidates coming out of Phase I trials and into Phase II. One is the vaccine developed by GSK mentioned previously, M72 + AS01E, currently enrolling adult participants in Phase IIB clinical trials in South Africa, Kenya, and Zambia. Another vaccine, Hybrid 4 + IC34, is entering Phase IIa clinical trials and is a partnership with two commercial entities, Sanofi and Valneva, the Danish vaccine and diagnostics research institution Statens Serum Institute, and Aeras. It is the first vaccine to be tested with a prevention-of-infection approach rather than prevention-of-disease, a new focus of TB vaccine research mentioned in the previous chapter as a potentially positive step because these trials can be shorter and smaller. Since rates of tuberculosis infection are always higher than rates of active disease, fewer people are needed to determine whether a vaccine candidate prevents infection. Duration is shorter because trial participants do not have to be followed for two years to see if they develop active tuberculosis symptoms (Frick 2015). An interesting point made by Mike Frick of TAG in his 2015 overview of tuberculosis vaccines is that the prevention-of-infection approach focuses on HIV-negative adolescents and adults rather than infants. Adults and adolescents, not children and infants, transmit the majority of tuberculosis globally in part because the latter typically have nonpulmonary forms of TB, which do not transmit through the air. Harking back to the discussion in the previous chapter of defining success in testing new therapies for diseases such as tuberculosis, an Aeras-funded study claimed that an adolescent or adult vaccine with only 40 percent efficacy would avert 70 percent of expected tuberculosis burden in low-income countries between 2024 and 2050 (Frick 2015).

Engaging, with Purpose

Driving the 112 kilometers from Cape Town to Worcester is a study in contrasts. Leaving the city, you pass on the right the comparatively prosperous and stunningly beautiful wine-growing area of Stellenbosch. Slightly further on you pass through the craggy Hawequas mountains, and soon after enter Worcester. Before I set out, a SATVI staff member had warned me not to be fooled by the pleasant middle-class homes visible at the western end of town; SATVI's clinic facilities were located further on, in the poorer neighborhoods supplying participants for the trials SATVI runs. For Aeras, SATVI, and TB Alliance, the unfortunate irony is that they require poverty and high rates of tuberculosis (and sometimes HIV) to conduct clinical trials, even while they are simultaneously seeking in the longer term to ameliorate what they require in the short term.

Worcester is an ideal site for conducting tuberculosis clinical trials for reasons having to do with geography, history, and government policies characterizing South Africa but relevant in some form to clinical trial sites in other low-income countries. Geographically, Worcester is close enough to Cape Town to enable principle investigators to commute back and forth as they conduct trials in Worcester while living in Cape Town. Second, about two-thirds of SATVI's staff either live in or are based at their Worcester site, including clinical researchers involved in recruitment and informed consent, nurses taking blood and conducting medical observations, and other medical staff (Hassan Mahomed, former director, Clinical Vaccine Trial Program, SATVI, personal communication, December 2, 2010). And finally, histories of colonialism and apartheid left majorities of Black and Coloured[2] South Africans in poverty. As Charles Feinstein notes in his economic history of South Africa, by 1994—the year apartheid ended—White incomes were almost nine times higher than Black incomes, and only Brazil had a higher rate of income inequality (2005). Postapartheid economic policies have done relatively little to ameliorate continuing race-based disparities in vital statistics, access to resources, and employment. Nor have they mitigated suboptimal living conditions for the many South Africans living in extreme poverty. According to the 2011 census, 86.6 percent of all households living with no income were Black, versus only 7.1 percent of White households; the lowest income category comprised 92.3 percent Blacks versus 2.9 percent Whites. Female-headed households constituted over half of low-income households. Though Blacks did make substantial gains in middle-income households from

2001 to 2011, there was virtually no decrease in the proportion of Blacks in the low-income or no-income categories (www.statssa.gov.za).

Though relatively small at a population of 78,906, Worcester is a microcosm of South Africa in the demographics outlined above. Based on 2011 census counts, Coloured and Black constituencies make up 72 percent and 8.7 percent, respectively, of Worcester's population, with Whites making up the majority of the rest at just over 17 percent. Over half of the population has only some secondary schooling or less, and 36.3 percent of households are headed by females. Though data is not disaggregated by racial category, more than one-third of households live on 38,200 South African Rands or less compared to the average of 201,339 Rands for South Africa as a whole and, more starkly, compared to the 2 percent of households in Worcester living on 614,000–2,457,600 South African Rands a year. Almost 9 percent of households in Worcester have no income at all (www.statssa.gov.za). The last statistic of note is that as of 2006, the area of Worcester where trial recruitment takes place had a reported all-tuberculosis rate of a staggering 1,400/100,000 (Mahomed et al. 2011). Overall rates found among 6,363 Worcester adolescents in a study to find tuberculosis incidence were a lower but still disheartening 200/100,000. All of the cases found were Black or Coloured, and not surprisingly, those living in poverty were at greatest risk (Mahomed et al. 2013).

On the other hand, postapartheid health-care mandates have improved access to health care, made primary care in the public sector free, and evidenced more hospital and clinic construction (A. Neely, assistant professor of geography, Dartmouth College, personal communication, June 2, 2014). SATVI uses a modest but well-equipped clinic in Worcester where the mothers are recruited and the babies who are enrolled in clinical trials get checkups and follow-up exams. A small but similarly well-equipped hospital is next door for those babies that present with signs of tuberculosis, and close by is a large provincial tuberculosis hospital, Brewelskloof, that primarily treats MDR-TB. According to the hospital's superintendent, Dr. Danie Theron, everyone in the Western Cape (the province in which Worcester and Cape Town are located) has access to HIV and tuberculosis treatment, and the hospital itself does not suffer from a shortage of drugs for their patients (personal communication, March 24, 2011).

It is the political economic contours of poverty and disease that are unfortunately key to why Worcester became and remains a clinical trial site apart from its clinic, pharmaceutical, and staff infrastructures. The bottom line is that researchers need high densities of tuberculosis to effectively conduct clinical trials for tuberculosis therapies; the lower the density, the more participants are required to be able to achieve any kind of meaningful results. Farming and migrant labor are common in the province, meaning high levels of rural poverty and for the latter, a difficulty in diagnosing, treating, and tracking individuals with TB. South Africa emphasizes Directly Observed Therapy, Short-course (DOTS), for those with tuberculosis, an approach where health-care workers go to patients and observe them taking their drug regimens. It is widely regarded as beneficial in aiding the completion of drug treatment, yet this also becomes much more challenging and expensive in the rural areas surrounding Worcester where those with TB can be far apart and far from clinic facilities.

The province's MDR-TB surged in 2007, an outcome Theron thinks was in part due to a bad batch of rifampicin, one of the four drugs constituting first-line tuberculosis drug regimens. It could possibly be traced to a bad batch discovered in 2002 after the manufacturer made what they described as a minor formulation change in their rifampicin, but were not required to submit updated bioavailability data. Bioavailability is the degree to which the active ingredient in a drug—that is, the component of a drug that works against the targeted disease—gets absorbed into the bloodstream. Bioavailability testing of single drugs, as opposed to FDCs, is not required in South Africa, thus the defective batch was only found after testing 118 patients at Brewelskloof Hospital revealed the low rifampicin levels (McIlleron et al. 2002). Though the Depot (the government drug supply center) subsequently switched back to an earlier manufacturer, such instances point not only to challenges in drug supply but to persistent problems of both substandard and falsified drugs in many parts of Africa and beyond. Substandard drugs in particular—that is, those that actually contain the active ingredients stated on the label but (typically) in smaller quantities than indicated—are playing a role in creating patterns of resistance to infectious diseases, as well as increased morbidity and mortality (Peterson 2014; Newton et al. 2014).

Tuberculosis is also not adequately tested and diagnosed in the province given large rural areas where mobile clinics are likely to come by once a month—not nearly sufficient, according to Theron, to detect TB and get patients into treatment before infections spread. According to Paul Spiller, a physician and administrator working at the Cape Town–based Brooklyn Chest Hospital, insufficient numbers of GeneXperts also contribute to problems finding and treating more individuals with TB.

GeneXperts are the recently developed diagnostic machines capable of assessing accurate diagnoses not only of tuberculosis but of drug-resistant tuberculosis within two hours, rather than the two or more weeks typical of other methods. This in turn promises to lose fewer patients to follow-up and to identify more MDR patients and get them on second-line drug regimens at early stages of the disease. Insufficient numbers of machines, however, means having to send sputum samples off to the nearest machine in another hospital, adding days to the results and in the process losing numerous patients to follow-up who cannot afford to return to the clinic a second time (Spiller, personal communication, March 25, 2013).

Coinfection with HIV has also surged: from 30 percent of those female patients hospitalized in Worcester for TB in 2008, to 70–80 percent three years later; and for males, a surge from 5–10 percent to 60 percent (Theron, personal communication, March 24, 2011). By the time these individuals come to the hospital, their CD4 counts are often as low as 20; the normal range is between 600 and 1,500. Had they been diagnosed earlier they would likely not have tuberculosis, much less be acutely ill with other opportunistic infections (Theron, personal communication, March 24, 2011). Confirming that his hospital also often does not see tuberculosis patients until they are acutely ill, Spiller added that economics and stigma largely explain why: individuals are reluctant, or simply unable, to seek medical care until their tuberculosis is far advanced. The risk of income loss, as well as discrimination from neighbors or employers, is too great (personal communication, March 25, 2013).

Finally, the TB hospital sees children with MDR-TB in addition to adult patients. As Theron noted, some of these children come from conditions of such acute deprivation they are remitted to foster care when released (personal communication, March 24, 2011). Part of the reasoning behind this drastic move is because typically MDR-TB patients are released from hospital after six months, even though they have eighteen or more months left of a complicated drug regimen involving fifteen to twenty tablets. Side effects are common and often extreme as well. Taking the two issues together, remaining on this regimen can be extraordinarily difficult, especially for children whose parents might be unable to assist or supervise because of work schedules (Theron, personal communication, March 24, 2011). The right amount and kinds of food also help with tolerating the regimen, and as Theron noted, this can be given to the children while in hospital; once they are out, it is not at all assumed that they stay adequately nourished (personal communication, March 24, 2011). Whether or not foster care is the right decision, it highlights the collisions of political, material, and scientific environments of tuberculosis evident in Worcester and its surrounding environs: namely, that even successfully treating individuals' tuberculosis becomes a potentially temporary proposition when their everyday living conditions are conducive to bacterial proliferation; that children with multidrug-resistant strains of the bacteria are the most poignant and damning signs of long-standing government and industrial neglect; and that current MDR treatments generate their own set of profound personal distress and logistical challenges.

These factors, in addition to a general lack of pediatric dosing in current TB drugs, explain why tuberculosis in children is becoming more central in discussions of priorities within the tuberculosis research community. For Worcester as a whole, the conditions and contexts described above all converge to explain why there is only a 35 percent cure rate for MDR-TB patients at Brewelskloof Hospital (Theron, personal communication, March 24, 2011)—a rate that is unfortunately not uncommon in other regions of acute deprivation and disease burdens.

Juxtapositions of poverty and expertise, material deprivation, and medical infrastructure are unfortunate necessities yet insufficient measures of a potential clinical trial site—at least for PDPs. Another key element for PDPs, as opposed to most industry-sponsored trials, is to determine whether particular communities actually want new vaccines and want trials being conducted in their communities. As noted by Lew Barker, senior medical advisor for Aeras, when Aeras first went to South Africa they held a town hall–style meeting to determine the level of political will behind getting a new tuberculosis vaccine. And that, noted Barker, was over ten years ago. And, he added, that needs to happen with every community they work in if trials are going to be successful in recruiting and retaining participants, and if participants are going to be convinced that their country and community will be beneficiaries of any successful product tested. All of the countries Aeras is working in now, including Kenya, Uganda, Senegal, Gambia, Mozambique, Cambodia, and India, are countries that want a better TB vaccine and are willing to participate in the effort to get there (Barker, personal communication, October 15, 2010).

Gaining a thumbs up on political will leads to the next two steps in turning a community into a trial site: as suggested by Suzanne Verver, senior epidemiologist for the KNCV Foundation,[3] the first step is to conduct basic epidemiological studies determining whether rates of tuberculosis in various age groups are high enough, and if so, getting a sense of how easy it is to enroll and retain individuals for studies (personal communication, November 15, 2010; Mahomed, personal communication, December 2, 2010; Willingham, personal communication, June 16, 2010). Being able to follow patients over relatively long periods of time is particularly important in tuberculosis clinical trials given the length of follow-up periods.

To that end two preliminary trials examining aspects of the BCG vaccine were run between 2001 and 2006, enrolling a total of twelve thousand infants. Another trial was run on adolescents, following them over the course of two years to test not only levels of tuberculosis but immune responses in those developing TB versus those who did not (Willem Hanekom, former codirector, SATVI, personal communication, February 7, 2011). There is little doubt that qualifying on the first count—more than adequate levels of tuberculosis to recommend clinical trials—related to qualifying on the second: community members ready to sign themselves or their babies up for trials. Only then was Worcester transformed from an impoverished community suffering sky-high rates of tuberculosis to an internationally recognized and respected clinical trial site. In fact for a while the Worcester site was the only tuberculosis clinical trial location. Even other high-burden countries often do not have the concentration of tuberculosis needed to make late-stage clinical trials feasible. This, combined with lack of adequate infrastructure and inadequate funding to develop necessary infrastructure and expertise, has made it difficult until more recently to plan multisite tuberculosis clinical trials. Despite the REMox trial failure, one of the beneficial achievements was improving clinical facilities and training staff to meet GCP standards across trial sites, as well as enhancing laboratory capacity so that there are multiple microbiology labs able to participate in large clinical trials (www.tballiance.org).

Ironically, going into communities and doing baseline epidemiological surveys itself jeopardizes the further possibilities of clinical trials, if for the right reasons. As you find cases, Verver noted, you treat them, and then there is less transmission, and ultimately lower incidence rates (personal communication, November 15, 2010). The contingent ethics of tuberculosis clinical trials thus is apparent even before they get started: the point of these trials of course is eventually to ameliorate burdens of tuberculosis, but doing so is contingent upon first capitalizing on those same burdens. Treating cases as they are found, though the ethical thing to do and the practice followed by SATVI and others, jeopardizes the possibility of conducting clinical trials and subsequently of preventing much larger numbers of tuberculosis cases.

For Worcester, the next stage of site development was training various staff for clinical trial support. As explained by Marijke Geldenhuys, former professional development and quality control manager for SATVI, training needed to start from the ground up given that most of the staff at Worcester came from the community and did not have research backgrounds. A first step was realizing that the more everyone knew about tuberculosis and about clinical trials, the better everyone could do their particular jobs and understand how these fit within the broader picture of clinical trial process and function. So, with the initial support of Aeras, Geldenhuys developed an approach to training that brought everyone regardless of background to the same approximate knowledge level. Whether individuals were drivers, cleaners, or investigators, starting in 2003 they went through the same basic course on tuberculosis, HIV, and malaria (the main infectious diseases in South Africa), the history of clinical research, where GCP came from, and how everyone fit together in the broader clinical trial enterprise. Given that some staff such as recruiters would have to explain concepts such as randomized trials or incidence rates of tuberculosis, other modules such as biostatistics and epidemiology were added as well (Geldenhuys, personal communication, April 6, 2011). This model of across-the-board staff training was then used by Aeras in developing sites in other countries like Kenya, answering concerns of standardization but also acknowledging that theirs was a successful and—according to Geldenhuys—relatively unique model of clinical trial site development (personal communication, April 6, 2011).

Visual materials developed by staff are essential components of recruitment. Posters advertising the current clinical trials were printed in Afrikaans, Xhosa, and English and hung around the clinic, and a comic book called *Carina's Choice* was also written by SATVI staff with the advice of community members and the very active CAB liaising between SATVI and trial participants. Meant as an educational outreach as well as a recruitment tool, the book talks about the extent and symptoms of tuberculosis, why a more effective TB vaccine is needed, and why clinical trials are necessary and participation essential to trial success. It was also written in the relevant languages and emphasized pictures with pared-down text in order to accommodate variable education levels. The booklet in this case is aimed more specifically at bringing recalcitrant men on board, given SATVI's experience that mothers are more apt to understand the risks of tuberculosis and to enroll their infants into a clinical trial than are fathers (Amit Makan, communications coordinator, SATVI, personal communication, March 24, 2011). The comic book subsequently was distributed to schools as well as other community venues, and more recently was transcribed into a play and performed at several high schools in the Cape Town area (Tameris 2014).

Explaining the details of tuberculosis and the necessity for testing is commendable, and *Carina's Choice* is doing a community service by reaching multiple demographics including adolescents. Most people are all too aware of the existence of tuberculosis and its devastation in and around Worcester, but not all know the details of symptoms or want to get tested. It is evident, however, that the book is nevertheless geared primarily toward recruitment. Education happens in the midst of the main story line featuring a SATVI nurse approaching a young woman sitting in the waiting area of a clinic with her baby. The nurse begins telling the woman, Carina, about what SATVI does and why, explaining the function of vaccines, the inadequate protection of the current BCG vaccine, and the process of vaccine trials. The point is made very clearly that finding a more successful vaccine was critical to ridding the community of tuberculosis. Clinical trials, then, become vital to intervening in a preventable disease that is devastating the Worcester community. And since this book was geared toward the MVA85A trial, it in turn meant that enrolling infants became a necessary part of that promissory endeavor.

The hope of tools like *Carina's Choice* is that relations of trust can strengthen once more community members know about SATVI and the work that they do. The book even takes steps toward addressing fears of potential participants by posting the trial participant Bill of Rights on the back, making clear that everyone has a right to information or to exit the trial at any point once enrolled. Yet recruitment is still a meticulous and time-consuming endeavor. For the MVA85A trial, mothers were found from birth registers the clinical team had permission to access. From there, team members went to the homes of these mothers, where they asked them if they could tell their story of the vaccine trial, accompanied by pictures. If mothers said they were willing to enroll their babies, then the team members thoroughly went through a sixteen-page consent form in the relevant language—typically Xhosa or Afrikaans. Enrolled babies, who were typically only two- to three-weeks-old, were usually followed for one month before actually giving them the vaccine, to make sure the baby was truly healthy and on a good growth trajectory.

Babies who passed this one-month screening were put at eighteen to twenty-four weeks in the experimental arm and given the BCG vaccine and then MVA85A as a booster, or placed in the control arm and given just the BCG vaccine, which is the standard for all babies in South Africa. The mothers brought their babies to the clinic facilities to receive vaccines, where they also had opportunity to ask further questions of nurses. The babies were followed up on days seven, twenty-eight, and eighty-four, with SATVI workers going to babies' homes to weigh, check on general health, and determine if someone else in the house had active tuberculosis or if the baby was showing any signs or symptoms of TB. If they did show signs, they were taken to the on-site hospital facility where they were tested and, if positive, were started on treatment. The babies were followed for a total of two years to determine signs of tuberculosis after vaccination (Michele Tameris, principle investigator, SATVI, personal communication, March 24, 2011).

Divisions of labor in clinical trials are well defined, and following GCP, all practices are well documented. As with academic and commercial clinical trials (see DeBruin, Liaschenko, and Fisher 2011), principle investigators are responsible, among other things, for meeting the recruitment quota as specified by trial protocol, while staff are more responsible for auxiliary everyday issues in clinical trial roll out. Nurses drew blood for analysis, while clinical research workers managed documentation, informed consent, fetching mothers, carrying equipment, labeling tubes, and other tasks (Tameris, personal communication, March 24, 2011). It was Geldenhuys and her staff who identified and addressed many of the issues including informed consent and recruitment procedures that needed attention and, sometimes, improvement. As she suggested, there is an almost bewildering array of tasks and skills involved in running clinical trials, and constant oversight is necessary to insure that all of these tasks—from data collection and analysis, laboratory work, machine calibrations, paperwork, patient follow up, and much more—remain up to GCP standards (Geldenhuys, personal communication, April 6, 2011). This training would need to happen at any clinical trial site meeting GCP standards, but at sites like Worcester, the long-term effects on job conduct of chronic personnel and resource shortages have to be undone as well. As a principle investigator working on tuberculosis drug trials put it, people are used to cutting corners in order to triage and do the best they can with not enough (Diacon, personal communication, March 25, 2011). What in everyday clinic practice is an unfortunate necessity in the context of resource deprivation becomes a liability in the context of a clinical trial meeting ICH guidelines.

The last thing to mention here about Aeras and SATVI's engagement in trial communities is the key role played by their CAB. CABs have become a staple of especially noncommercial clinical trials; they are required to be a part of trial protocol for example in NIH grants. But in previous studies I have done interviewing researchers involved in AIDS vaccine clinical trials, it became clear to me that CABs were not especially vital to the process of clinical trial design and conduct. They seemed to exist more in name than substance. This is not true of the CAB that acts as a very active liaison for SATVI between researchers and trial community members. They come from numerous sectors of Worcester society, from community leaders to nurses to individuals who believe in what SATVI is doing and want to play a role. They actively perform outreach and tuberculosis education for community members, dispelling myths about what researchers are there to do and what trials are about. But they also bring concerns and questions from the community to researchers and advise on how to approach particular issues and misunderstandings. Their role is critical in forwarding fears and desires to researchers who otherwise might not be available to hear these or be unaware that they exist. CABs, in other words, when they are utilized to the fullest are able to bridge to at least some extent the considerable divide between two highly unequal constituencies.

TB Alliance is also heavily involved in community engagement where they conduct clinical trials. They also develop TB educational outreach materials and programs, and they have CABs that are very much like SATVI's and Aeras's in playing key communication and navigational roles before and in the course of clinical trials. TB Alliance also sponsors regionally specific workshops on tuberculosis, training on TB drug research, education and awareness campaigns, and broad-scale surveys determining what countries want in terms of the therapies themselves, their delivery methods, physician attitudes toward incorporating new regimens into their practices, National Tuberculosis Program capabilities in implementing new regimens, and purchasing mechanisms that might be necessary (TB Alliance 2009).

Engagement by TB Alliance, Aeras, and SATVI is considerable and is taken seriously. They go a distance in determining the will of communities for new therapies and for hosting clinical trials, and they conscientiously educate about early signs of the disease, the need for testing and treatment, and modes of transmission. The bottom line of this engagement, however, is recruitment. This does not erase the good that these organizations do; it means that in order to conduct the clinical trials they need to conduct, they have to get community members on board with their objective. As TB Alliance says on its website, "without informed and engaged communities, the development and delivery of new and improved TB cures is not possible" (www.tballiance.org). The broader reach of trials, their prequels, and their sequels in other words is, as Kelly and Biesel state it for malaria eradication projects (2011, 73), "a better way to connect landscapes of innovation with landscapes of well being."

It strongly evidences that despite the contexts of inequality characterizing trial sites, potential trial communities have significant power in determining whether they participate or not in clinical testing and with what caveats of trust and communication. Achieving the goal for recruitment into MVA85A took a long time, for example; mothers were not at all sure they wanted to enroll their infants into a medical experiment. On the other hand, as more studies are suggesting, when community members hear about a new therapy that is meant for them and addresses a health problem they care about, they feel like they are part of the solution when they participate in trials (Engel et al. 2014; Zvonareva and Engel 2014; Stadler, Delany, and Mntambo 2008). Communications from the CAB also force researchers to address alternative understandings, objections, and fears of potential participants. Though the response might be to attempt further awareness through a biomedical lens, there is nevertheless a degree to which researchers become privy to the different roles therapies play in communities before and during trials, variant modes of understanding and treating disease, and the location of tuberculosis within community priorities (Stadler and Saethre 2011).

Parameters on Clinical Trial Design

The purpose of GCP rules in ensuring standards for clinical trial design and conduct are a clear response to trials occurring across regions and countries and to increased focus on drug and vaccine safety. Yet for tuberculosis trials, these rules can generate tensions between what is dictated by regulatory parameters for standardized data collection versus what is humane practice especially in the context of entrenched poverty. These tensions can take many forms, but they typically stem from the everyday realities of individuals who might be un- or underemployed, whose wages are inadequate, and who can be undernourished or food insecure. For many individuals in these circumstances, enrolling in a clinical trial can at least assure them good medical care. An example of where parameters of these trials can preclude the neediest—that is, those who perhaps need clinical trials the most—comes in an exchange between the principle investigators of the MVA85A trial and another tuberculosis researcher. The principle investigators had published an article in the British medical journal *The Lancet* discussing the trial, including the methods and basic criteria they used for recruiting the infants. The researcher who was invited to respond to this article pointed out that the investigator and her colleagues had not mentioned environmental factors, including malnutrition, in the development of tuberculosis and in responses to a vaccine. Malnourished individuals, the author goes on to say, have shown compromised T-helper (immune) cell response in TB. In fact, given the strength of this association according to the author, giving children enough nutrition would reduce tuberculosis perhaps more than the vaccine (Upadhyay 2013).

The investigators' response was to say that all the babies enrolled in the trial were given multivitamin and iron supplements for two months before and one month after the trial and that infants were referred during follow-up for nutritional support or to health services if they showed signs of failure to thrive. They also mentioned that acutely ill or clinically malnourished infants were excluded from enrolling in the trial (Tameris et al. 2013). These comments are illuminating on a number of levels. They illustrate the degree to which clinical trials, even those within the humanitarian pharmaceutical model, are designed as highly controlled environments that do not necessarily mirror the more precarious environments of the communities in which they are embedded. The phrase that babies needing nutritional support were referred "during follow-up" also signals the regimentation of trial design and practice: nutritional supplements typically would not be given during a trial because this would be considered an intervention—that is, something that could cause a change in vaccine response. Nutritional supplements would be given to the experimental arm if the point were to test improved response to the vaccine with better nutrition. Interventions other than the one being tested—in this case, a vaccine—are thus carefully avoided, and if they occur can ostensibly muddle the integrity of data being collected and threaten FDA approval. And finally, clinically malnourished babies are rejected as trial participants because of safety reasons, not wanting to jeopardize the life of an immune-compromised child. They are also rejected because healthy babies make better data: the commentator is correct in saying that malnutrition can change immune responses to vaccines just as nutritional supplements can, and this is exactly what the investigators don't want.

Similar tensions characterize international ethical guidelines on informed consent and local variations in knowledge systems, health literacies, and decision making. As an increasing number of scholars are suggesting, the concept of informed consent as enshrined in the Helsinki Declaration and other medical research ethics guidelines is one that assumes particular conditions of autonomy and self-governance. While holding onto the overall point of trial subject safety, scholars are increasingly seeing informed consent documents as cultural artifacts: products of particular modes of thinking and of liberal notions of individuality and rational behavior. As Sariola and Simpson suggest, there is then assumed to be a "seamless diffusion of ethics" to all international clinical trial settings (2011, 519). If the purpose of informed consent as an ethical tool is to protect participants and to ensure as far as possible that coercion and misunderstanding play no role in recruitment, many scholars and researchers argue that approaches to informed consent practices need reexamining (see Miller and Boulton 2007; Frimpong-Mansoh 2008; Tindana, Kass, and Akweongo 2006; Gikonyo et al. 2008). Gikonyo and colleagues make several suggestions, including seeking permission from community heads before approaching individuals, considering informed consent a process rather than a singular event, and periodically assessing understanding through questionnaires during the course of the trial (2008). The problem is that the FDA and EMA have not made changes in their regulatory policies governing informed consent practices to allow for regional contexts, and until this happens, trials testing new therapies for eventual approval will maintain their practices accordingly.

There are examples in which context-specific informed consent practices are being followed, but they are not the norm. Tindana and colleagues, for example, state that a regional health research center in Ghana has for years followed local rules, including approaching chiefs first to ask permission to conduct a health intervention before proceeding to get individual consent (2006). These are locally driven interventions, however. Of note about much of this literature is that the hierarchies and gendered politics of localized decision-making structures are not under scrutiny: that community heads are in many areas likely to be men, who would then be giving permission for women or children to participate in trials, for example, is not questioned. The point is to interrogate the rigidity of current informed consent practices and to make them visible as culturally embedded.

Under these regulatory confines, however, SATVI has been attuned to the histories, social dynamics, politics, and economies mediating what it takes and what it means to be a human subject. As Geldenhuys describes the process at SATVI, they attempt to link informed consent to something that is meaningful to community members through relevant examples, language geared to local expressions, or understandings of health and illness. In so doing, the team situates what can become an empty if not counterproductive standardized tool of ethical research into a relevant context of experience and understanding. So when community staff receive new protocols they take them point by point to figure out how best to explain different concepts to potential recruits, incorporating both role-playing into the training process and different materials such as pictures into the educational outreach, recruitment, and consent processes. These careful considerations were meant to more adequately convey to trial participants the structures and parameters of clinical trials, especially those facets such as randomization and double-blind control and experimental arms that are especially difficult to translate into localized structures of meaning (Geldenhuys, personal communication, April 6, 2011). The consent form stands at sixteen pages and contains a prolific amount of information, but the question still has to be raised of how much participants understand of what they are or are not undertaking. Despite the important discussions ongoing about the form and function of informed consent, no one has resolved the difficulty of conveying into localized rubrics of understanding concepts that are foreign to just about anyone outside of biomedicine.

Other parameters of clinical trial design and implementation unrelated to GCP requirements became apparent at a Community Engagement workshop at the 2013 Union World Conference on Lung Health in Paris. A senior researcher for SATVI, for example, pointed out that sometimes sponsors (including Aeras) gave clinical trial protocols—the formal blueprint for trial design and conduct—to SATVI with only a few weeks to finalize them, making meaningful feedback from SATVI researchers or community members next to impossible. Sponsors' obligations to other stakeholders including journals can also skew facets of trial conduct including the notification process. In the case of the MVA85A trial, for example, results first had to be published in the British medical journal

The Lancet before trial participants were allowed to know that the trial had failed (Tameris 2013). TB researchers also expressed frustration that community members and the CABs that represented them were not being adequately drawn into the actual design of clinical trials but rather were asked to communicate concerns after trials were implemented (Hamilton 2013).

These frustrations were aimed at tuberculosis research as a whole, not specifically at TB Alliance or Aeras. Yet what they describe are not just shortcomings in community engagement efforts, but the various and sometimes unexpected obstacles delimiting efforts to include participants well in the research process. The frustrations were widespread enough that a September 2015 workshop called the Combined Community Engagement Forum, sponsored by TB Alliance and two other global health organizations, International AIDS Vaccine Initiative (IAVI) and AIDS Vaccine Advocacy Coalition (AVAC), took place in South Africa with the agenda of ratcheting up efforts to improve community participation in clinical trials. The workshop included eighty tuberculosis and HIV researchers and community members and began with the recognition that efforts in community engagement had not yet had much impact on research communities. The next step was making stakeholders equal partners and thinking deeply about strategizing more encompassing and meaningful approaches to community participation. Obviously one workshop does not galvanize all the changes needed, but it was a start and one that will hopefully generate more workshops and more meaningful action in the near future (CPTR 2015).

The points discussed above suggest a broad spectrum of issues facing TB Alliance and Aeras as they negotiate the social order of clinical trials and the larger distributive, financial, and individual logics of which they are a part. The tensions between strict requirements of international clinical trials, and more nuanced practices attuned to local understandings and politics, are difficult to resolve. Inflexible definitions of gold standard scientific evidence as enshrined in RCTs mean that researchers especially in resource-deprived areas are at times forced to put data integrity before the overall welfare of participants. It even sometimes means, as the respondent above pointed out, not delivering interventions that ironically would help the very disease being addressed. It thus potentially stretches the distance between efficacies proven under trial condition and actual effectiveness of new therapies in populations. The distance, in other words, between laboratories and real bodies discussed by Barry (2005).

As with any encompassing and complex set of endeavors, there is acknowledged room for improvement in how Aeras and TB Alliance undertake research. As TB researchers themselves indicated, there is latitude even within acknowledged constraints to include community members in actual trial design and to include local researchers as full partners in protocol deliberation. There is undoubtedly an unequal balance of power between sponsor and host countries characterizing current clinical trial design and conduct, an inequality that could be mitigated with some changes in practice. These changes might in fact be coming soon. Charles Mgone, executive director of the EDCTP, outlined to me several areas where he is working to move EDCTP toward more equal African involvement in projects and to expand African-initiated research.

In the area of clinical trials, Mgone is advocating discussions by all partners, including local ones, regarding priorities for clinical trial design and for training that would make individuals across participating African countries employable not just in tuberculosis clinical trials but in other trials and scientific projects. Within and across African countries, Mgone also is supporting better networking among scientists at clinical trial sites. Rather than each trial site communicating with the European or American sponsor, as currently is often the norm, Mgone is moving toward communication networks among the participating trial site scientists. EDCTP also gives out networking grants to allow scientists to share data they are gathering, discuss problems or concerns, and exchange students or site monitors across countries and trial sites. And for the many scientists returning from abroad after earning PhDs, EDCTP offers grants for creating their own projects and research teams rather than working on northern-led projects (Mgone, personal communication, July 19, 2012). In the 2014 round of grant proposals, EDCTP has partnered with the WHO's Special Programme for Research and Training in Tropical Diseases (TDR) to fund scientists from sub-Saharan Africa and low- and middle-income countries, respectively, to be placed in pharmaceutical companies or PDPs for extra training in skills for conducting clinical trials (www.EDCTP.org).

Accounting for Benefits

Benefits to trial communities, as Hayden (2007) and others point out, also remain a complex if not fraught domain. What kinds of benefits, who ends up benefiting and how, and who controls benefits are all questions that remain difficult to resolve in the context of clinical trial inequalities. It is critically important—and highly commendable—that Aeras and TB Alliance promise new vaccines and drug regimens to those who need them including communities involved in proving them efficacious. Yet this promise is speculative in that it portends a reward in the distant future while capitalizing on individuals' bodies in the here and now; and it is high-risk speculation given how many therapies fail even in late-stage clinical trials. Indeed, so far success in realizing this promise has remained elusive. In a sad irony, as mentioned in the introduction, the only two tuberculosis drugs with new mechanisms of action to receive regulatory approval in the last forty years were developed by pharmaceutical companies, both of which have priced their respective drugs beyond the reach of most individuals living with tuberculosis.

Janssen's bedaquiline received limited approval by the FDA in 2012, while Otsuka Pharmaceuticals' delamanid received limited approval by the EMA in 2014, both after Phase IIb clinical trials. Limited approval is awarded with the understanding that the approved drugs will quickly enter Phase III trials for final testing of safety and efficacy. For both drugs, approval remains limited to those individuals with MDR-TB who have no other options, until both companies perform Phase III trials. Otsuka is moving forward with Phase III trials, but Janssen so far is not; Janssen on the other hand is registering bedaquiline in several low-income countries, but Otsuka is not following suit with delamanid: it has not registered delamanid in any high-burden country so far, including those countries where clinical trials were performed. Janssen has opened up some compassionate use programs where drugs such as bedaquiline that do not have final approval are nevertheless made available to those who have run out of treatment options; yet Otsuka has refused to do this until Phase III trials are conducted, even though compassionate use by definition aims at those with no other choices but to accept a higher level of risk in a treatment that has not been completely vetted for safety and efficacy (Lessem 2014a). Meanwhile, delamanid costs the equivalent of about $43 per pill in the UK, the only country other than Germany where it has been registered; while bedaquiline costs nearly $150 per pill in the United States, and nearly $5 in low-income countries (Lessem 2014a; 2014b). The uptake of both these medications, needless to say, has so far been marginal.

For community staff, benefits are more immediate since they are paid for the work they do during clinical trials. Yet as others have argued

(Checkley and McShane 2011), staff nevertheless occupy precarious roles. Clinical trials are on timelines: they might last for two years or so, but then they are over and so are paid staff positions. Several more trials are being or will be conducted at the Worcester site, but these will not necessarily occur without interruption. However, and in the meantime, it is expensive to continue paying staff in between trials, and funds are typically inadequate in tuberculosis research to cover times of hiatus (Checkley and McShane 2011; Tameris 2013). The individuals working at the Worcester trial site are not immune to these concerns, even though the training they receive at SATVI brings with it somewhat greater potential than staff at some trial sites for finding employment elsewhere. Training, however, is never the only consideration in searching for and acquiring new jobs; the cost of uprooting families, adjusting to new schools and communities, and moving away from the support of relatives are equally trenchant considerations. Yet the qualifications staff receive with their training are likely to mean that alternative jobs will be well outside of Worcester given the paucity of other clinics and laboratories.

The most obvious benefits to trial communities is the access to clinics, diagnostic technologies, laboratory facilities, and trained health personnel that exists as a direct outcome of clinical trials. While some health personnel as noted above will find employment elsewhere once clinical trials end, others will remain, to the benefit of the community and its immediate surroundings. Equipment brought by trial researchers stays at site locations even after trials end, making labs and clinical facilities better equipped than many—at least for as long as equipment remains functional. As Geissler et al. determined from surveying participants in clinical trials in Uganda, satisfaction from clinical trials was in part derived from the fact that clinics were closer, trained nurses were "right on the doorstep," and more medicines were actually stocked and available than was typical of government clinics (2008, 698).

The question remains how to multiply and sustain these positive aspects of clinical trial development after trial sponsors have relinquished responsibility. This is perhaps the most serious sticking point of including participants well: clinical trials are by default ephemeral phenomena. Even for Aeras and TB Alliance, like their commercial counterparts, the end of trials portends the loss of jobs and research opportunities and the likelihood that health care in trial communities will degrade as resources to support diagnostics, drug supplies, and expertise diminishes. Distinct from commercial trials, however, closing tuberculosis clinical trial sites hopefully signals an imminent arrival of better treatment and prevention and herein remains the promise of accountability for these PDPs.

The Reach of Research Ecologies

The efforts outlined above, despite their limitations, arguably move toward what Hayden calls "distributive agency" (2007), that is, the notion that benefits should not just flow to the more enfranchised, but to trial community populations as a whole. I want to extend the question of benefiting trial communities to address the very relevant argument that clinical trials create enclaves of better health care, biomedical resources, and employment opportunities within regions of widespread deprivation (Sparke 2014). A different but not entirely unrelated critique is that PDPs such as TB Alliance and Aeras focus too narrowly on technical rather than broad-based interventions (Buse and Harmer 2007; Buse and Walt 2000).

Rather than supporting or refuting these critiques, I want to complicate binaries of technical versus social and enclave versus broader geographic distribution of benefits accruing before, during, and after clinical trials run by TB Alliance, Aeras, and their institutional partners. Speaking first to technical versus social binaries, many scholars have made the argument already that drug regimens and vaccines are not simply technical interventions. Instead, they have "social lives" (Whyte, Van der Geest, and Hardon 2002) that always "go beyond the body, affecting and potentially reshaping interpersonal, family, and community domains" (Petryna, Lakoff, and Kleinman 2006, 8). PDPs like TB Alliance and Aeras recognize that the technologies already available for tuberculosis have particular and often negative impacts on those with or at risk of TB and their families. First-line drugs are tedious, inconvenient, and not always consistently available over the six to nine months they have to be taken. Second-line drugs for MDR-TB are highly toxic and prohibitively expensive and can exact enormous physical, emotional, and financial tolls on families as well as patients. Variable and often low levels of protection with the BCG vaccine mean that families in high-burden areas live with the knowledge that tuberculosis is a constant possibility for themselves and their children. Even in high-burden regions, stigma can still plague those with tuberculosis and their families; procuring drug regimens can be time-consuming, and in some regions expensive, adding extra burdens to other family members in the quotidian demands of household upkeep; and income loss from one, and sometimes more than one, family member incapacitated from tuberculosis can be devastating.

Critics of the technical fix thus often overlook the fact that particular drugs and vaccines already exist for specific diseases like tuberculosis, and that these can be causing multiple and deleterious social, financial, and psychological impacts on families. What TB Alliance and Aeras propose to do first and foremost is ameliorate these multiple impacts by improving upon the technologies. Critiques of technical interventions are most valid when they point to the disproportionate attention technological fixes receive in global health initiatives. There is no question that more funding needs to be channeled toward interventions into the many socioeconomic outcomes of poverty, but these need to complement, rather than displace, vaccine and drug development.

That Aeras and TB Alliance are considering a very broad array of upstream and downstream facets as part of the remit of vaccine and drug development also sets them apart. For their "What Countries Want" report, for example, TB Alliance conducted interviews of 222 individuals in five high-burden countries to ascertain what "improvement" would mean, for example, how important interaction with ARVs would be, optimal delivery methods (i.e., tablets or capsules versus injections), and the "key success factors" for adopting new regimens (TB Alliance 2009, 6). Though significant regional variations in responses pertained among interviewees in the five countries of China, India, Brazil, South Africa, and Kenya, TB Alliance confirmed that reducing treatment times was important to all constituencies, as was the compatibility of a new TB regimen with ARVs for coinfected patients (TB Alliance 2009, 10). For regulatory officials and physicians in Brazil, China, India, and South Africa, having clinical trials conducted in their own countries was a requirement for new regimen approval; and for those in Brazil, India, and Kenya, evidence of "real-world effectiveness" of new regimens—that is, how new regimens worked in tuberculosis patients outside of trial conditions—would also be a requirement for pilot-phase adoption of new regimens (TB Alliance 2009, 12–13).

These and other opinions gleaned from interviews continue to guide the criteria TB Alliance committees use to move particular regimens forward, or not, and to shape the discussions ongoing with regional regulatory authorities, national ministries of health, the WHO, and other agencies in preparation for future rollout and optimal adoption of successful new regimens. Like any tool, the report on "What Countries Want" has its shortcomings, the most evident of which is that only fourteen patients or patient advocates were interviewed out of the total of 222. No patients or patient advocates were interviewed in China or South Africa. Clearly, the emphasis for TB Alliance was an overview of regulatory and health sector requirements rather than consumer desires.

The report nevertheless illustrates the point that TB Alliance, and Aeras by extension, takes seriously the myriad roles drug regimens and vaccines will play in reshaping relations at every level of society in the countries where they will be adopted. They are well aware that simply producing drugs or vaccine candidates is useless—by themselves, they are simply biologic and molecular entities with no value. It is the achievement of getting new drugs or vaccines into relevant bodies on a large scale that turns them into life-saving technologies with ripple effects across the spectrum of material, social, and psychological arenas. This, in turn, requires attention to a complex range of logistical, regulatory, and financial factors as well as consumer desires. TB Alliance and Aeras, in conjunction with the WHO, the FDA, and purchasing agencies such as GAVI and UNICEF, are attempting to encompass most if not all of these factors, and in doing so they strengthen public health systems beyond tuberculosis or its attendant technologies.

Turning to the second point regarding enclaves, TB Alliance and Aeras's particular approach to therapeutic production and dissemination means that they produce agglomerative effects extending well beyond the enclaves of clinical trial communities. In addition to what has already been described, this includes strengthening regional regulatory agencies, evaluating public and private clinical capacities, negotiating technology transfers, and working with the WHO and other global agencies to better ensure consistent high-quality supply chains. Technology transfers are of course not unique to tuberculosis PDPs, or to PDPs at all. Like technology transfer agreements within the commercial pharmaceutical sector, PDP agreements benefit a fundamental agenda of getting drugs or vaccines more efficiently disseminated into particular geographic regions. The difference from industry agreements is that the ultimate goal is not about generating demand and expanding markets, but about adequately meeting long-standing need. As such, PDP agreements move toward enhancing capabilities of all partners, encompassing late-stage research and development, knowledge sharing, and scaled-up manufacturing.

One example of the add-on value of therapeutic production is TB Alliance's licensing agreements with both the Shanghai Fosun Pharmaceutical Development Company in China and its subsidiary, Shenyang Hongqi, and India's Open Source Drug Discovery Programme (OSDD) of the Council of Scientific and Industrial Research (CSIR). Fosun is a major health-care company in China, and Shenyang Hongqi is China's largest manufacturer of tuberculosis treatments (TB Alliance 2014b). CSIR is a government consortium of thirty-seven scientific laboratories, and OSDD is a consortium funded by the CSIR focusing on research and discovery of novel therapies for diseases including tuberculosis (TB Alliance 2013). Licenses for these entities concern the above-mentioned drug combination PaMZ. In these new agreements, BMGF and TB Alliance found a partial answer to persistent funding issues: both Fosun/Hongqi and CSIR/ OSDD will be conducting their own late-stage clinical trials within their respective registered territories of China, Taiwan, Hong Kong, Macau, and India. As emphasized by Derek Ambrosino (personal communication, October 7, 2014), these trials will not be part of STAND (Shortening Treatments by Advancing Novel Drugs); they will be conducted independently by Fosun and CSIR without subsidization by TB Alliance, though any data emerging from the trials will be shared. Should these trials prove successful in showing the efficacy of PaMZ for either or both drug-sensitive and drug-resistant tuberculosis, the licensing agreement includes a commitment to manufacture the drug regimen and make it available at affordable rates for the millions within those regions living with tuberculosis.

As Mel Spigelman, CEO of TB Alliance, stated in an April 2014 news release, this is "the sort of agreement that product development partnerships are able to achieve to benefit the millions of patients needlessly dying" from tuberculosis (TB Alliance 2014b). One facet making these agreements easier is the negligible IP transfer involved: by the time Phase III trials are over, Bayer's patent on moxifloxacin will have expired; pyrazinamide's patent has long since expired; and TB Alliance controls PA-824. This means no negotiations over pricing or distribution with commercial partners and facilitation of manufacturing and marketing in the event of a successful regimen. The agreements benefit all partners in other ways as well. TB Alliance gains a means of moving its regimen forward into expensive Phase III clinical trials, and potentially to the millions currently living with TB in India, China, and surrounding areas. China and India bolster their pharmaceutical consortia focused on infectious diseases and the downstream effects of infrastructure, education, jobs, and expansion of expertise into tuberculosis research. The licensing agreements brokered by TB Alliance include clauses, however, that ensure the work promised by all partners gets done. For both CSIR and Fosun, TB Alliance or another partner will step in should there be dissatisfaction about the mode or pace of progress (TB Alliance 2014b).

Trial site development itself also has effects beyond site communities that bear noting. As already mentioned, rigorously trained clinical trial staff have enhanced employability at other clinical facilities. The best evidence that Geldenhuys was accurate in claiming the appointability of SATVI staff is that several have been hired by other research organizations (Geldenhuys, personal communication, April 6, 2011). Benefits potentially accrue as well to scientists involved in clinical trials. Exchange programs have developed to bring scientists from African countries to UK or European universities to finish their PhDs, and vice versa (Gillespie, personal communication, July 30, 2013); and the EDCTP's efforts should begin to pay off in expanding opportunities for African scientists to be principle investigators in locally relevant and locally initiated trials.

New Ethical Questions

After all the discussion of clinical trials, a question remains over whether they should be taking place at all right now given the limitations on what we know about the tuberculosis bacterium. The arguments of those advocating for trials to continue are compelling: Can we wait until we have clear and adequate information about protective immune responses to the bacterium, or do we potentially save hundreds of thousands of lives with candidates currently in the pipeline? As Sally Merry notes in her work on the rise of indicators in, inter alia, health and human rights arenas, the "magic" of numbers comes in their ability to convert complicated and contextualized situations into clear and objective measures. While seeming open to public debate, they nonetheless present indisputable realities (Merry 2011). So for the argument that holding off on clinical trials would mean huge numbers of lives lost, while this is no doubt true, it nevertheless circumscribes the existence of perhaps better alternatives, while also obfuscating the much more complex realities behind those numbers. The numerical argument for continuing trials for four-month drug regimens, for example, is somewhat countered by one study that through computer modeling found there would be significant regional variation in reduction of tuberculosis mortality, incidence, and health-care expenditures as a result of shortened drug regimens (Dowdy 2014).

But other questions also arise. How many more lives could be saved with much shorter regimens (i.e., two weeks) or much more effective vaccines? Is continuing with clinical trials the most ethical thing to do when there is significant potential that those trials will fail until better understandings of the bacterium bring expanded capabilities of predicting success? Safety of trial participants is not so much in question since this aspect of new drug and vaccine candidates can be effectively tested. It is the good will, patience, and trust of trial communities that is in question, and whether they should be recruited into clinical trials that have less than optimal assurances of success.

Clearly the same question has been taken up by the primary funders of tuberculosis clinical trials. Though the NIH and the European Consortium have channeled resources into basic science research for tuberculosis all along, in 2014 BMGF made a shift in its funding allocations from clinical development to basic discovery, preclinical development, and Phase I studies (Frick 2015). The reasons for this are multiple. It becomes difficult to rationalize enormously expensive Phase III trials when failure rates are high; basic science will eventually uncover a biomarker for TB, enabling trials to be shorter; with deeper understandings of *M. tuberculosis* and the immune responses that protect the body against it comes improved predictability of which candidates will be effective; and in the case of vaccines, basic scientific research will facilitate the design of vaccines that can target the right antigens and trigger a broader range of immune responses. Right now, vaccine candidates are targeting only 12 out of a total of 4,500 possible antigens in the *M. tuberculosis* genome, and they focus almost exclusively on triggering T cell, or cell-mediated, responses in the immune system rather than antibodies produced by B cells, or what is called humoral immune responses. As summarized by Mike Frick of TAG, "the antigenic repertoire targeted by vaccines in the pipeline is narrow, overlapping, and aimed at a single arm of the immune system" (2015).

It remains true that even a marginally effective vaccine administered globally to one hundred million individuals will save hundreds of thousands if not millions of lives. Similarly, a four-month drug regimen potentially means hundreds of thousands more individuals can complete their treatments, that millions of dollars will be saved in reduced costs, and that untold cases of MDR-TB will be averted by increasing adherence rates. Yet what might those numbers look like if the money currently expended on later-phase clinical trials was directed instead toward basic science? And what if those expanded resources galvanized within only a few years the ability to conduct much shorter and smaller trials that are far more predictive of success? And that the new candidates derived from deeper understandings of *M. tuberculosis* had far higher efficacy rates and significantly shorter treatment times? Those numbers are even harder to argue with. Equally important, it is hard to argue with the implications for future clinical trials and their many participants.

Conclusion

Like their commercial counterparts, the tuberculosis vaccine and drug trials discussed in this chapter are complex and dynamic sites at the center of ongoing debates over the form and function of medical research. Ethical debates in particular have become more strident in the face of recent trends of pharmaceutical companies conducting trials in low-income settings, yet rarely registering new drugs in the countries where they test them. Perhaps the only positive to come out of this trend is that the increased scrutiny has broken the Möbius-strip nature of previous ethical debates over what constitutes an "ethical trial" in different geographic settings. Instead of endless rounds arguing what it means to shield human subjects from harm, and whether the answer to this question depends on where the trial is, scholars are stepping back and asking a much broader spectrum of questions about benefit sharing, engagement, capacity building, and enhancement of well-being.

My aim in this chapter has been to join these scholars in asking questions that treat tuberculosis trials not as static and delimited entities, but rather as highly dynamic, contingent, and sometimes contradictory processes. I also take as a given that every trial is a thick entanglement of social inequalities, contrasting knowledge systems, institutional structures, scientific dictates, colonial histories, postcolonial politics, and bacterial parameters. Yet this does not mean that all trials are the same, and there are ways that tuberculosis PDPs approach trials that make a significant and positive difference. One of those is that they locate trials in low-income regions because that is where the overwhelming majority of individuals with tuberculosis live, not because these populations are more exploitable and potentially expendable.

There is little question, too, that the trials run by tuberculosis PDPs like TB Alliance and Aeras and their partners such as SATVI make earnest attempts to include participants well: through their early and ongoing community engagement, CABs, educational outreach programs, and meticulous approaches toward informed consent, trial communities move closer to being active arbiters of scientific practice at the same time many become champions of the technologies they are helping to produce. Indeed the MVA85A participants were not unusual in feeling they had done something "for the benefit of the community as a whole and for future generations" as a character in *Carina's Choice* says. Though the vaccine in that trial failed, participants wanted to know when the next one was so they could sign up again (Tameris 2013). Other studies of clinical trial participants—those who participate in trials targeting diseases or products relevant to trial communities—suggest similar findings that the social value of the research and the chance to play an integral role in ridding country and community of infectious disease were critical in decisions to enroll (Akrong, Horstman, and Arhinful 2014; Zvonareva and Engel 2014).

Communities benefit from training programs, research opportunities, and well-equipped clinics. The flow is not entirely one way, however: communities play an important political role in determining whether a research site will be located in their midst and whether the ultimate agenda of producing new therapies is tenable or taking the appropriate form. Community members are also able, primarily through the CAB, to communicate dislikes, hesitancies, and misunderstandings, or even to share alternative understandings of research and therapeutic efficacy.

The broader reach of TB Alliance, Aeras, and SATVI's approach to conducting clinical trials adds to the constellation of factors making these therapies positively different from their commercial counterparts. Once again they diverge significantly from the underlying motivations and practices of commercial trials and encompass governmental, community, and regulatory relations not replicated in commercial endeavors. Equally important to note is that tuberculosis trials are generating important discussions within the research communities and the organizations that support them. These discussions revolve around how to enable potential trial participants more say in designing clinical trials, how to strengthen local research capabilities and locally determined research projects, and how to realign institutional demands of notification and protocol. All of these potentially mobilize critical changes to trial procedures as they point to the examined and unexamined assumptions embedded within RCTs and their ever-changing social order (Marks 1997).

Discussions also continue to be productive, even if so far they are irresolvable, around regulatory requirements for strict standardization within clinical trials that can collide with the highly diverse range of social practices, nutritional levels, comorbidities, understandings about health and disease, and even the specific coordinates of deprivation across trial sites. At the heart of this disjuncture is a question about what "scientific integrity" means when the sources of data production are human bodies invariably possessing molecular and physiological variations that cannot be filtered out by strict qualification criteria. Is it better science to continue attempts to homogenize the bodies constituting clinical trials so that data is more pure, which in turn leads to more clear-cut regulatory approval decisions? Or is it better science to lessen the distance between the "aseptic laboratory" and the "intertwined humanities" (Bensaude-Vincent and Stengers 1996, 263) that will ultimately constitute the beneficiaries of new tuberculosis therapies? Focusing on the latter might strike a better balance between understanding clinical trials as highly controlled scientific experiments exporting laboratory-like conditions to the field and seeing them as a hybrid of standardization and flexible adaptation to regional social and somatic variance. There is an argument to be made, after all, that regulatory approval should incorporate realities pertaining on the ground in the interests of enhancing post-marketing effectiveness of drugs and vaccines. So far, this is not the current trajectory of clinical trials, and yet the FDA as a site of governance has shown itself to be adaptive to changing scientific and political contingencies.

That inequalities are required by researchers working hard to find technical solutions to a particular facet of poverty leads to a greater messiness characterizing tuberculosis clinical trials. Messy because participants on the one hand are consultants, advocates, active agents, and future consumers of new therapies, but at the same time—like their counterparts in commercial trials staged in low-income regions—their constrained access to health care and acute levels of deprivation inform in profound ways not only why clinical trials move into their communities but why individuals decide to enroll in them. Yet once participants have enrolled, SATVI, Aeras, and TB Alliance make earnest efforts to include them well within these constraining regulatory parameters. They remember why they are there and what the ultimate goal is of the complex and contingent endeavors they manage. It is this remembering for whom and for what purpose that must remain at the heart of how tuberculosis trials are envisioned, designed, and deployed.

CONCLUSION

Tuberculosis and the Future of Humanitarian

Pharmaceutical Production

After reading an earlier draft of this book, one reviewer commented that I was telling two stories: one about tuberculosis, and the other about PDPs. The recommendation was that I focus my attention on the PDPs. This book *is* largely about PDPs, but by default it also has to be about tuberculosis; the two are inextricable. First, because tuberculosis PDPs in some respects function differently than other PDPs given the particularities of the tuberculosis bacterium. But second, there would be no tuberculosis PDPs if better treatments and vaccines had already been developed; if the neglect of global health agencies, departments of health, and governments over the decades had not paved the way for tuberculosis to sustain its presence; and if the worst inequities of late twentieth- and early twenty-first-century global capitalism had not given tuberculosis fertile grounds to thrive, including in its close association with HIV infection.

The question raised in the introduction of why tuberculosis only recently has been made a matter of urgency in new global health initiatives should really be a question of why it took so long, and why much of the world collectively turned attention away from a disease that never ceased its devastation. Accordingly, people involved in the PDPs I have highlighted in this book do what they do not because they wanted to work for a PDP per se, but because they wanted to do something about tuberculosis. PDPs were either the places to be able to do the work they wanted to do and believed in or they were the key organizations with which to partner. Gérald Voss, head of GSK's vaccines for developing countries unit, even said with a wry smile that there was no shortage of scientists wanting to work in his unit rather than elsewhere at GSK (personal communication, July 6, 2012).

Writing about PDPs in this book has also been something of a tale of two phenomena, though: tuberculosis PDPs as initiatives emerging from new global health priorities and focused on tackling a single disease with new technologies, and PDPs as alternative models of pharmaceutical production diametrically opposed to the mainstream pharmaceutical industry in addressing global health need rather than market incentive or shareholder demand. This book is about the latter. Its main goal is to make PDPs visible in a way they haven't been before: as scientifically, politically, and socially innovative models of pharmaceutical development, or what I am calling humanitarian pharmaceutical production.

In fact, the therapies PDPs develop are distinct products altogether from their commercial counterparts because they are not just different in developing therapies for diseases the pharmaceutical industry has ignored. Their divergence is encompassing: from their philosophical foundations to their approach to science, poverty, the communities they target, and the procedures for achieving their goal. Their departure begins from the knowledge that the pharmaceutical industry has failed to account for the majority of the world's disease burdens. From there, tuberculosis PDPs turn the incentives for pharmaceutical development around, tackling a disease that affects more people than almost any other, but people who are overwhelmingly poor. In other words, they take burdens of disease rather than shareholder demands as the bottom line of what kinds of new drugs and vaccines should be developed. With this revised mission, in turn, comes both the onus and opportunity to think differently about what researching and developing new therapies should be about, the set of relations it should encompass, and the practices it should champion.

Accordingly, tuberculosis PDPs have mobilized a whole constellation of regulatory, consumer, governmental, scientific, and financial relations that are different from, or nonexistent in, pharmaceutical industry production. TB Alliance and Aeras retool patents to protect pharmaceutical discoveries from overt commercialization so that their therapies can stay low cost, and they are both seeking new mechanisms of finance that will sustain if not enhance their budgets and thus their portfolios of new therapies. They advocate for regulatory reforms that can shorten time to approval of new drug regimens, and they attend in their research and development processes to the best balance of cost and effectiveness. They have expanded significantly the remit of what it means to produce drugs and vaccines, from FDA or EMA approval and marketing to working with governments, purchasing agencies, ministries of health, potential consumers, the WHO, and physicians to ensure new therapies actually get to the people who need them. They have initiated new ways of doing science in valorizing the productivity of open knowledge exchange across scientific disciplines and diseases and in recognizing the creative potential in failure. In order to test new therapies, they seek the will and approval of potential trial communities, design outreach programs and educational workshops, and engage in local capacity building.

PDPs like TB Alliance and Aeras tell us not just what is possible but what is desirable in reenvisioning the goals pharmaceutical development should be achieving and for whom. They disrupt complacency toward what has become normative—that is, that pharmaceuticals are developed for all those who can afford them, rather than all those who need them. They go toward answering James Ferguson's provocation of whether we might "find ways of thinking creatively about the progressive possibilities . . . of this new terrain of transnational organization of funds, energies, and affect" (2010, 169). The nonlucrative pharmaceuticals PDPs are developing in essence broadcast the political message that everyone's lives should matter and that the market is not always the right tool for ensuring even minimally equitable social benefits.

To the extent that I have focused on PDPs as components of global health initiatives, it has been to suggest an alternative thinking to the dichotomizing critiques arguing against technical fixes as misguided, and for social and economic interventions as the antidotes truly needed in solving disease burdens of the poor. To this argument are three counterarguments. First, that the approach tuberculosis PDPs use in their alternative models of therapeutic development include community engagement, public health strengthening, enhancement of pharmaceutical purchasing and implementation, and local capacity building in terms of both professional training and infrastructural development. They are not, in other words, just technical fixes. The work they do in ensuring that any successful new vaccines or drug regimens get where they are needed and wanted means going well beyond the laboratory into social, economic, geographic, and political arenas of action.

Second, arguments against technical fixes create false dichotomies that not only narrowly categorize approaches as technical or nontechnical, but pit these approaches against each other rather than recognizing how they work together to be mutually beneficial. There should be no question that more effective vaccines and shorter, simpler treatments are needed for tuberculosis. Vaccines have played a vitally important role in diminishing many infectious disease burdens, and an effective tuberculosis vaccine could similarly be critical to reducing transmission and disease. Providing a much shorter, simpler regimen to those millions already suffering from tuberculosis and enduring long, arduous, and in the case of MDR-TB, expensive and highly toxic drug regimens also is critical, and humane. Having said this, preventing people from getting tuberculosis or curing them if they have it does not put food on the table or create jobs where currently there are none. As Randall Packard said long ago in his masterful history of tuberculosis in South Africa (1989), a disease of poverty like tuberculosis cannot be entirely vanquished until political economies of exploitation, discrimination, and deprivation are themselves overturned. Global health initiatives are also targeting the social and economic conditions fostering the poverty that in turn breeds tuberculosis, but these in turn will work best when deployed alongside efforts toward therapeutic improvements.

This, however, segues into the third argument, which is that any and all kinds of global health initiatives stand much less chance of success in the face of ongoing facets of the global economy that perpetuate gross inequalities within and between countries and increase the breadth and severity of poverty. With the end of the era of Millennium Development Goals in 2015, the UN has now declared a set of Sustainable Development Goals that call for ending poverty, ensuring well-being for all, and promoting inclusive economic growth, among other things (sustainabledevelop ment.un.org). However commendable these goals might be in theory, they will make little headway when UN-based global trade and IP policies continue to generate inequitable access to food, medicines, and other essential commodities, and when bilateral trade agreements perpetuate other kinds of global inequalities including low-wage jobs and lax oversight of workplace conditions. UN agencies need to work in conjunction with each other, not at cross-purposes, and governments in turn need to rethink policies and regulations that undermine the health initiatives they simultaneously support with millions of dollars in annual aid donations.

These other necessities raise the point that pharmaceutical humanitarianism by itself cannot achieve justice for the communities they are serving. Though reducing tuberculosis burdens would play a significant role in restoring economic capabilities as well as individual morale, it will not, alone, rectify other social, political, and economic injustices the poor typically endure. Only when taking all of these facets together—new therapies, significant social and economic gains in regions of resource deprivation, more equitable global economic policies—would pharmaceutical humanitarianism be part of restoring justice to those they are trying very hard to make healthy. Nevertheless, going ahead with what tuberculosis PDPs are doing is critical. To not continue to act even in the face of inaction in the other two fields would, recalling Paul Farmer (2004), simply be compounding injustices.

PDPs, too, are not the only alternative to commercial pharmaceutical production. Other initiatives have been implemented, or are ongoing, that aim to redress those areas of pharmaceutical need ignored by the pharmaceutical industry (Nathan 2007). There are other PDP models like the Drugs for Neglected Diseases initiative (DNDi), for example, that also work toward developing pharmaceuticals for neglected infectious diseases. DNDi works somewhat differently than the tuberculosis PDPs highlighted in this book: it steers away from BMGF funding and relies instead on government and individual donations and some industry subsidizations; its founding members include European and Malaysian, Kenyan, Indian, and Brazilian institutions, creating greater geopolitical equity in expertise and knowledge exchange; and it focuses more heavily on South–South technology transfers, using pharmaceutical companies in participating countries where possible. Yet in the field of malaria, for example, DNDi focused its attention on repurposing already existing drugs, successfully rolling out two FDCs utilizing three already existing malaria drugs. This is a significant achievement as it simplified treatment and addressed the problem of drug resistance in two different high-burden regions (Craddock 2015). Nevertheless, it also targeted an area of pharmaceutical development requiring much less expense and time because drugs were used that already existed. Redressing pharmaceutical need does not always lend itself to these expediencies: for tuberculosis, existing antibiotics can possibly be repurposed and used for tuberculosis treatment, but new drugs with novel mechanisms of action are also needed. With other diseases, drugs do not always exist for repurposing. DNDi's model as a whole is not replicable, then, though many of their approaches are commendable and should be replicated where possible.

An alternative tactic to PDPs is incentive systems to prod pharmaceutical companies or any innovator to focus attention on drugs for poor populations. One of these is the Health Impact Fund (HIF), a proposed international agency funded through pooled government contributions raised through income taxes. Companies or innovators could then register new products with the HIF in return for agreeing to sell them globally for ten years at a price no higher than the cost to produce them. In return, they would receive for those ten years funds from the pool proportional to the health impacts actually achieved by the new product (Pogge and Hollis 2011). Again, this concept has much to recommend it: as Pogge and Hollis explain (2011, 331), the use of taxes to fund the HIF means spreading the onus of responsibility widely and therefore thinly; they calculate that coming up with the $6 billion needed for the HIF would mean something less than a 0.01 percent increase in average tax rates in high-income countries.

But the problem with the HIF financial incentive is that it would not be anywhere near proportional to the profits pharmaceutical companies make from other means. Individual innovators might be enthusiastic, but they would likely be unable to manufacture any new product at a scale needed for global distribution. So far, governments have not been keen to pay into funds that work differently but toward similar ends—like the Global Fund, which is perpetually underfunded and begging for countries to fulfill their promised allocations. In the United States, too, even a very small income tax increase that would go for foreign assistance would be highly controversial and unlikely to pass. And deciding upon and enforcing criteria for what constitutes the nature and degrees of health impacts would be mired in politics and delays. Finally, $6 billion is nowhere near adequate to meet current pharmaceutical need in low-resourced regions; to come anywhere close to meeting that need, multiple times that amount would be necessary.

A new initiative recommended by the WHO and hosted by UNICEF, the United Nations Development Programme, the World Bank, and the WHO Special Programme for Research and Training in Tropical Diseases (TDR), called the International Fund for R&D, resembles the Global Fund. It will be constituted by donating governments as well as those impacted by infectious disease burdens; funds from participating governments will be pooled, and a committee will select proposals from low-income countries needing subsidization of research and development for technologies to address their health needs (Moon 2014). Once proposals are selected, the International Fund will orchestrate their implementation, and a scientific advisory committee will also be formed. Open innovation approaches will be emphasized, and contributions especially from emerging economies will be encouraged (Moon 2014). Like the Global Fund, the International Fund could make headway in getting a number of projects moving forward and in ensuring that innovations happened within low-resourced countries and in ways that make sense for target populations and regions. Yet, a global organization run by several high-level global health and research organizations might get bogged down in bureaucracy, losing efficiency and effectiveness. Like the Global Fund, the International Fund would almost certainly be plagued by inadequate contributions from member governments, and in fact, in essentially creating competition with the Global Fund, the problem of contribution shortages would likely be exacerbated.

A final example is using legislation such as the U.S. Orphan Drug Act of 1983 as a different kind of incentive to address neglected areas of pharmaceutical development. Orphan drugs refer to drugs for diseases that are relatively rare in occurrence and thus typically have no or inadequate drugs to treat them because of an insufficient market base. The Orphan Drug Act thus provides incentives such as tax breaks and fast-tracking FDA regulatory approval for drugs developed for diseases falling within the orphan category. Yet as Peter Arno and coauthors describe, the act has had relatively little impact on drug development for diseases actually rare in occurrence. Rather, it has aided pharmaceutical companies who have been able to successfully interpret the act to include crossover diseases such as AIDS as an orphan disease, thereby benefiting from the incentives provided while developing drugs that would bring them millions in profits anyway (Arno, Bonuck, and Davis 1995). This is a good indication that any legislation with similar incentives for neglected disease development would face the same consequence of outcomes that were unintended and unhelpful to anyone but pharmaceutical companies.

All of these initiatives have strong advantages as well as limits. What they all signal, however, is that currently the pharmaceutical industry works for a severely delimited strata of people living in high-income regions, rather than the majority of the world. Some of the initiatives attempt to redress this problem through independent or government bodies that circumvent participation of large Western pharmaceutical companies; or they attempt redress directly through pharmaceutical companies, but with rewards rather than regulation. In some respects, the tuberculosis PDPs highlighted in this book come the closest to reforming the pharmaceutical industry from the inside: they insist that industry partners play by bottom-line rules of affordability and access, even though this is not always enforceable; they turn infectious disease research into market opportunities through emerging economy partnerships and creative financing mechanisms; and they are demonstrating even to pharmaceutical industry executives that scientific innovations are more likely to emerge from PDP models of open knowledge exchange, scientific creativity, and cross-institutional and cross-disciplinary collaboration.

Yet, three pharmaceutical companies have exited tuberculosis research and development in three years, and two other companies— Otsuka and Janssen—are treating their new tuberculosis drugs like any other, with high prices and limited distribution. A recent Memorandum of Understanding between the U.S. Agency for International Development (USAID) and Janssen to make bedaquiline (brand name Sirturo) available at no cost to low-income populations is evidence that community pressure can result in compromises on the part of pharmaceutical companies. The compromise in this case, however, deserves very limited commendation: Janssen has only agreed to donate $30 million worth of bedaquiline over four years, or a total of thirty thousand treatment courses (Stop TB Partnership 2014a). Given the profound need for lower-cost drugs for those with MDR-TB, and the equally profound lack of better and more affordable alternatives, this measure is unacceptable. It is the worst kind of band-aid measure affording Janssen some reprieve from public castigation while actually doing little to ameliorate the plight of more than half a million people.

The challenges faced in deploying new technologies in regions characterized by extensive resource deprivation can also not be understated, which is one reason TB Alliance and Aeras are doing predeployment research in the countries they are targeting for new therapies. A new diagnostic technology provides a case in point. Diagnosis of tuberculosis is another area of long-standing neglect, with no improvements for decades over older and less than optimal methods for diagnosing drug-susceptible TB, as well as MDR-TB and those coinfected with HIV. Smear microscopy and solid or liquid culturing, the two most common diagnostic tools, are either not particularly accurate, cannot diagnose drug susceptibility, have biosafety concerns, or have protracted wait times of two to three weeks for results. In the case of even short lag times, there can be a significant problem of patient follow-up given the distances some patients travel to access clinic facilities. Returning a second time for a test result can be prohibitively difficult, resulting in individuals with newly diagnosed tuberculosis—drug sensitive or otherwise—not starting on treatment regimens and often not even knowing their diagnosis.

But then a few years ago came a breakthrough, the diagnostic tool GeneXpert that generated understandable excitement in the tuberculosis research and treatment community. Developed jointly by a diagnostics PDP, Foundation for Innovative New Diagnostics (FIND), and the California-based biotech company Cepheid, GeneXpert was developed in 2008 and received WHO endorsement in 2010 (www.finddx.org). In many ways, this new tool is exactly what the TB community has been asking for: it is fast, with results within ninety minutes; it is comparatively accurate; it can diagnose drug-resistant TB by testing for susceptibility to rifampicin; it requires very little training to use given that it is fully automated; it functions well even at higher ambient temperatures; and it requires no special biosafety measures. With FIND negotiating a 75 percent reduction on Cepheid's price of the machine, it also is relatively affordable at $17,000. With subsidies from BMGF and others, the assay needed for conducting tests with the machine cost $10 (Weyer 2012). By 2012, 33 percent of high-burden countries had ordered the GeneXpert including India, China, and several African countries (Weyer 2012; Gilpin 2011).

Despite the excitement over GeneXpert and the potential it holds for better and quicker diagnoses of tuberculosis, it has encountered problems. Technological innovations are rarely timed to coordinate with each other or with other facets of the larger context in which they operate. In this case the capacity of GeneXpert to diagnose accurately more individuals with TB, including MDR-TB and those coinfected with HIV, has run up against insufficient drug availability in many regions. There are consequently now lists of people in some places who have been diagnosed with rifampicin resistance but who cannot begin appropriate treatment because second-line drugs are not available (Weyer 2012). Even before GeneXpert was introduced, clinicians pointed out the problem many countries had in providing sufficient hospital beds, or enough beds with robust infection control in place, to accommodate MDR-TB patients. This problem, too, will only grow worse as more MDR-TB patients are diagnosed (Keshavjee 2010).[1] Even promising new technologies cannot be effective, and in fact can create extra problems, when operating within suboptimal environments lacking necessary corollary resources.

Further problems with GeneXpert are cost, space, and electricity supplies. Though the machine itself has been negotiated down to a more affordable level, actually utilizing the new technology is much more expensive. The full cost of rolling out GeneXpert for a year, including personnel, electricity, and assay cartridges, is more like $100,000 according to one WHO official (Gilpin 2011). As explained further at a conference poster session, GeneXpert also requires air conditioning despite the temperature range it tolerates, as well as steady electricity supplies and multiple outlets. With any fluctuation in electricity, data is lost entirely, and new samples need to be reobtained from patients. And though GeneXpert is meant for midlevel rather than local adoption, photographs in the poster showed a regional laboratory housed in an old rail car, evidencing the suboptimal conditions pertaining even at midlevel in many low-income countries. These conditions, in turn, make it challenging to incorporate GeneXpert technology even though it was designed to be space-efficient (Emenyonu Emmanuel, personal communication, November 12, 2012).

It would be easy to say that the story of GeneXpert suggests the need for the various PDPs to better coordinate the rollout of their technologies. Unfortunately, the reality is that technological development happens within variant time frames, making such coordination unfeasible. Despite the issues it has faced, GeneXpert is helping more people find out that they have tuberculosis and what kind, and many are starting the treatments they need. Starting treatment early means reducing transmission as well as getting more people healthy. But for those who are not able to begin treatment because of drug shortages, GeneXpert is making even more visible why new, simpler, and less expensive drug regimens are critically needed, including those that are compatible with ARVs for those with HIV coinfection.

Nevertheless, two presentations at the 2014 Union World Conference on Lung Health discussed flatlined funding levels for tuberculosis R&D and continuing resource inadequacies for drug, vaccine, and diagnostic development (Daniels 2014; Balasegaram 2014). At the same time, recent meetings among ministers of all the BRICS countries resulted in agreements to pool resources for tuberculosis interventions, including an aim to get 90 percent of their vulnerable populations tested for tuberculosis and those testing positive onto appropriate treatment (Stop TB Partnership 2014b). This is a very positive step. It responds to the desires of both Aeras and TB Alliance, among others, to galvanize these countries into more action on two fronts: doing more to address severe burdens of tuberculosis in their own countries; and mobilizing their considerable expertise and pharmaceutical infrastructure into tuberculosis pharmaceutical research and production. As elaborated in previous chapters, Aeras and TB Alliance would like to further the involvement of BRICS countries by having them commit resources for new drug and vaccine development; partnerships with China signal the beginning of this trajectory. Ultimately, the aim is to scale up production of resulting tuberculosis pharmaceuticals so that each BRICS country could become a regional manufacturer and supplier of quality tuberculosis drugs and vaccines.

Such a shift could go some distance toward addressing two limits to PDPs: their dependency on philanthropic donations and unreliable Western pharmaceutical partnerships; and their geopolitical inequality in resource flows and scientific exchange. PDPs currently still remain precarious financially, but they are becoming increasingly creative in their financing mechanisms and approaches. It makes sense for Brazil, Russia, India, China, and South Africa to play increasingly important roles in those approaches: together, these countries account for the majority of the world's tuberculosis, but they also possess abundant expertise, pharmaceutical infrastructure, and a regional economic presence. Tapping these countries' expertise and financial resources provides TB Alliance and Aeras alternative funding to achieve their goal of new tuberculosis drugs and vaccines, as well as enhanced scientific and manufacturing capabilities. BRICS countries, meanwhile, gain partners possessing an abundance of experience in tuberculosis research and the chance to address a disease important to their populations.

All or most of these countries, in addition to robust biomedical and biotechnology sectors, also have significant resources to commit to the tuberculosis research and development process. What this means is that they would more likely act as equal partners rather than subsidiaries to Aeras and TB Alliance, taking the lead as China is doing in assuming responsibility for research and testing procedures. Indeed, in the case of China, at least, TB Alliance and Aeras are showing the way to what might be Phase II of tuberculosis PDPs: working as equal partners with countries to coproduce new therapies. Along with technology transfers could come upstream and downstream benefits, but with the difference that host countries could take the lead in public health strengthening and directing progression of research and development. BRICS countries could also lead the way in forging more robust and efficient regional regulatory agencies, while also potentially formulating norms and requirements better suited to regional economic, social, and political contexts.

Partnerships with other BRICS countries will not look the same as current partnerships with China, but the opportunities are there to continue the best of the humanitarian pharmaceutical production model, while redressing current limitations and shortcomings. Such an expansion of pharmaceutical development that meets the needs of countries' populations, however poor, symbolizes a victory not just for those suffering from tuberculosis. It could provide hope for those millions suffering other diseases having no or inadequate treatment, while evidencing the global economic and social benefits of addressing the health of all rather than the few. It could demonstrate the incalculable gains, in other words, of making the humanitarian pharmaceutical production model the norm rather than the exception.

ACKNOWLEDGMENTS

THE RESEARCH FOR THIS BOOK would not have been possible without a generous grant from the National Science Foundation (STS/SES Grant 1027285). It allowed me to travel to conferences, trial sites, and pharmaceutical production facilities; to interview dozens of people; to hire research assistants; and to have a year's sabbatical in which to research and begin writing the book. During my sabbatical, Jean-Paul Gaudillière generously provided me an office at the Centre de Recherche Médecine, Sciences, Santé, Santé Mentale, et Société (CERMES3), as well as his invaluable advice on my project and on the presentations I gave at CERMES3, Le Londe les Maures, and Paris.

I have benefited exponentially from the questions and comments of the many participants at the workshops, colloquia, and conferences where I presented aspects of my research during the past several years; I cannot list all of them, but I hope they know I am grateful. I can at least thank those who invited me to the following venues: Gerry Kearns for the invitation to the "Vital Geographies" workshop, Cambridge University; Matt Sparke for the invitation to speak at the Department of Geography Colloquium Series, University of Washington, Seattle, and for his thoughtful comments and conversations on aspects of my work, and Katharyne Mitchell and Matt for their generosity in hosting me while in Seattle; Catherine Campbell, Flora Cornish, and Morten Skovdal for their invitation to the "Community Impact of Global Movements in HIV/AIDS" workshop, the London School of Economics; Jean-Paul Gaudillière for the Régulation, Norms et Saviors dans les Champs de la Santé Mentale seminar series, CERMES3, and for the European Science Foundation Program at CERMES3 and the École des Hautes Études en Sciences Sociales,

Paris; Iris Borowy for the "Government of Techno-Science, Technological Productions, and the Environment at Global Level" workshop, Le Londe les Maures, France; Deb DeBruin for the Center for Bioethics Colloquium series, University of Minnesota; Tamara Giles-Vernick for the workshop "Interventions in Whose Interest? African Health Issues from Multidisciplinary Perspectives," Fifty-fifth Annual African Studies Association Meeting, Philadelphia; Reg Kunzel for the Department of Gender, Women, and Sexuality Studies Colloquium Series, University of Minnesota; Vincanne Adams and Tobias Rees for the "Gateskeeping: Global Health and the Gates Foundation" workshop, University of California, San Francisco; Ken Waters for the Center for the Philosophy of Science Colloquium Series, University of Minnesota; and Seth Brotherton and Simon Reid-Henry for the "Counter Vitalities" workshop, Yale University.

I thank those who commented on my work, particularly Patricia Kangori and Salla Sariola, at the Pharmaceutical Life Cycle conference, Ziebergen, The Netherlands, 2013; to those at the "Making Scientific Capacity in Africa" workshop, Cambridge University, 2014; and to those, especially Vinh-Kim Nguyen, at the International Bioethics and Global Health conference, Oxford University, 2015.

Tamara Giles-Vernick, Regina Kunzel, Abby Neely, Rachel Schurman, Dominique Tobbell, and Vincanne Adams all agreed to read at least one chapter, and Dominique, Vincanne, and Abby read the entire manuscript. I owe a huge debt of gratitude for their wonderful comments both substantive and editorial. To Tamara I owe bounteous thanks for introducing me to colleagues at the Pasteur Institute and for her unending patience in listening to me. Fortunately, at least this last was often over a glass of wine. To my anonymous reviewers, I am in debt for the insightful comments, perceptive questions, and helpful suggestions. My book is a better one for the generosity of time and intellect of all my readers. Jason Weidemann was a wonderful, astute, and supportive editor throughout, and I am grateful that he made the process as painless as possible. To my fabulous former graduate student and research assistant, now a professor, Yeonbo Jeong, a huge thanks for the transcriptions of interviews and conference proceedings, and for the moral support and intellectual conversation over the years. Thanks also to Deborah Oosterhouse for the astute and meticulous copyediting.

To all of the people who agreed to speak with me about their work and organizations, I owe endless thanks. I never stopped being surprised at how readily these incredibly busy scientists, public health officials, staff, philanthropic representatives, and researchers gave their time to me, and how patient they were in explaining scientific concepts and processes. Many of these individuals also read relevant sections of the manuscript for accuracy, thereby giving even more of their time. I learned enormous amounts from their comments and can only hope that I have been able to do justice to their work and to their expertise. In this category many thanks go to Ann Ginsberg, David McCown, David Barros-Aguirre, Kari Stoever, Helen McShane, Stephen Gillespie, and Tom Evans. Carl Nathan also generously read a chapter of the manuscript, and his thorough comments and corrections were invaluable. Daniel Hoft of Saint Louis University and Fred Quinn of the University of Georgia stood in Amsterdam's Schiphol airport as we waited for our connecting flights on the way home from a conference and explained numerous aspects of their work on tuberculosis vaccines. Most of all, a huge thanks goes to Derek Ambrosino, formerly of TB Alliance, and Jamie Rosen, formerly of Aeras. As my main contacts at these organizations, they provided initial information, opened the door to other interviews, double-checked particular questions, read drafts of relevant chapters, and made sure others at TB Alliance, Aeras, and SATVI read drafts for accuracy. Jamie also arranged a tour of Aeras's offices and vaccine production facility.

Without my friends and family providing all kinds of support and just being there, this book would not have materialized. I owe all of them more than thanks. To the best staff in the world: Jenny, LeeAnne, Margie, Andrea, and Kayleen, thank you for cheerfully holding down the fort while I buried myself in revisions. You're all pretty great! To Jennifer Gunn, for weekends up north and dinners that are always balm to my soul. To Leslie Appelbaum, for the wisdom and comfort that come from knowing me forever and for always being there even if it means getting on a plane. To Darby Bonomi, for the trips through the years, the insights, and being able to have fun even when lost in the woods. To my partner David, for bringing so much laughter and love into my life, and for cheering me through the writing process. To my son Simon, who always reminds me what matters, keeps my perspective, and makes my heart swell. To my sister Elaine, who like all the best sisters has been there always, but especially when I needed it the most. And most of all to my father, Lane, who has not let a day go by in the past six years without asking about my book, assuaging my frustrations, commending my progress, boosting my confidence, and generally showing his abiding faith in me. Words are not adequate to express what that has meant to me.

NOTES

Introduction

1. Chemical libraries are facilities containing compounds developed by scientists as possible targets against particular diseases, but which proved ineffective in that capacity. The same compounds, however, could prove effective targets against other diseases, including tuberculosis. Though universities often have chemical libraries, they take up space and are expensive to maintain. Pharmaceutical company libraries are thus often superior resources, potentially containing hundreds of thousands of well-maintained compounds ready to be tested against diseases other than those for which they were originally developed.

2. The therapeutic revolution is widely defined as the introduction of sulfa drugs in the mid-1930s, the development of penicillin in the 1940s, the discovery of cortisone in 1949, and in the 1950s and 1960s the development of vaccines against polio, mumps, rubella, and measles, as well as oral contraceptives, antipsychotics, and tranquilizers (Tobbell 2012; Temin 1980).

3. As Mowery et al. (2001) note, the evidence of inadequate commercialization of federally owned patents rested on the very small percentage of 28,000–30,000 government patents actually commercialized. Yet most of these patents had been ceded to the government by private Defense Department contractors who had rights under pre-Bayh-Dole policies to retain patents but had not invoked these rights.

4. Thomas McKeown's study showed for populations in Britain that improvements in nutrition, housing, and other social factors predating antibiotics played more important roles in diminishing morbidity and mortality from infectious diseases including tuberculosis. The introduction of penicillin, according to McKeown's graphs, had less effect. The rise of HIV/TB comorbidities starting in the 1980s somewhat complicates this relationship, but

poverty is still a factor not only in HIV transmission but in tuberculosis as a primary opportunistic infection among people living with AIDS.

5. Me-too drugs are those compounds essentially the same as already patented drugs, but simply differing in delivery method, packaging, or dose. They are not characterized by any kind of therapeutic advance.

6. The actual cost of developing a new drug is highly controversial and varies depending on whom you talk to. Not surprisingly, 2006 industry estimates of $1.32 billion to develop a new drug are higher than industry watchdog figures or those of scholars who keep track of such issues. For a good critique of R&D costs as well as of industry arguments for needing to charge high drug prices in order to maintain R&D, see Light and Warburton 2011. Whatever the actual figure, what is agreed is that developing a new drug is extraordinarily expensive, and getting more so.

1. The Possibilities and Parameters of Drug and Vaccine Partnerships

1. As of June 2015, however, the German biopharmaceuticals company IDT Biologika acquired Aeras's manufacturing facility in a partnership designed to strengthen the capacities of both organizations for developing and manufacturing new vaccines (Aeras 2015).

2. Efficacy signifies a new therapy proving effective under controlled clinical trial conditions. It will only prove effective after use in wider populations.

3. Moxifloxacin is still used to treat tuberculosis, however. Like other drugs of its class, fluoroquinolones, it is used "off-label," that is, for an indication that it was not originally tested or approved for but for which clinical evidence suggests effectiveness.

4. As of April 2016, however, researchers at Oxford University who have also partnered with Aeras on vaccine trials announced the finding that a particular kind of T cell when activated was associated with higher risk of TB in both infants and adolescents, and that another particular T cell when activated was associated with lower risk of TB. These results, though tentative and needing further study, do suggest directions for scientists designing TB vaccines (Fletcher et al. 2016).

5. It is "almost" because some individuals with MDR-TB are also resistant to pyrazinamide, meaning that BPaZ would not be effective for these patients.

6. Stoever is not looking toward U.S. banks because, as she noted, they are less likely to embrace the social missions or accept lower rates of return.

2. Scientific Collaboration, Innovation, and Contradiction

1. New chemical entities are applications that come upstream of NDAs. They represent molecular compounds showing promise as potentially effective against particular diseases.

2. A new molecular entity is defined as "an active ingredient that has never been marketed . . . in any form" (Light and Lexchin 2012, e4348).

3. Ever-greening involves extending patents on drugs through minor alterations to the molecular compound, delivery method, or appearance that typically do nothing to improve therapeutic performance. Because it is an obvious way to maintain profits without actual innovation, it remains a controversial practice.

4. The obvious exception to this statement is the palliative therapeutics also produced by pharmaceutical companies in part as a redress to this contradiction—drugs for chronic diseases such as hypertension, diabetes, asthma, epilepsy, or AIDS, for example, are for the most part taken for the duration of a person's life. I thank Dr. Carl Nathan for this point.

5. Thank you to Carl Nathan for clarifying this process for me.

6. GAVI, the Vaccine Alliance, formerly the Global Alliance for Vaccine and Immunization, is a public–private organization combining UN departments, vaccine manufacturers, researchers, and philanthropists. It also is largely funded by BMGF, and its mission is to create "equal access to new and underused vaccines for children living in the world's poorest countries" (www.gavi.org).

7. The statistic of more cases averted than number of children is because over the course of forty-eight months, many children in the control group that did not receive RTS,S experienced more than one episode of malaria. Needless to say, this attests to the debilitatingly high rates of malaria in these regions.

8. Primary infection indicates initial infection with *M. tuberculosis* as opposed to reactivation of previous infections.

9. At the time of my interview in 2012, this machine had a price tag of $750,000, preventing Aeras from purchasing a machine with higher biomarker-detecting capacity (Graves, personal communication, June 6, 2012). By 2014, the price had dropped to $400,000. However, the cost of the machine is only one factor; the cost of assays and time associated with data analysis is also added, a cost that rises as the complexity of assays increases. Thank you to Andrew Graves for this update and clarification.

3. The Contingent Ethics of Tuberculosis Clinical Trials

1. Jill Fisher, however, makes a similar argument for clinical trials in the United States, where individuals enroll in trials because they have no other access to medical care (2007). Thanks to Dominique Tobbell for pointing this out to me.

2. "Coloured" is the term used in South Africa for people of mixed European and African or Asian ancestry.

3. KNCV is a Dutch-based international TB nonprofit organization.

Conclusion

1. There are pilot programs in some countries that both shorten treatment for MDR-TB to nine months or a year and also do away with the need for hospitalizing patients. These, however, are not yet standard practice (Van Deun 2012; Kuaban 2012).

BIBLIOGRAPHY

Adams, Vincanne. 2013. "Evidence based global public health: subjects, profits, erasures." In J. Biehl and A. Petryna, eds., *When People Come First: Critical Studies in Global Health*, 54–90. Princeton, NJ: Princeton University Press.

Aditama, Tjandra Yoga. 2011. "Building partnerships for supporting scale-up of the drug resistant TB program and strengthening second-line medicine management in Indonesia." Session on Strengthening Partnerships for Pharmaceutical and Laboratory Care, 42nd Union World Conference on Lung Health, Lille, France, October 27.

Aeras. 2015. "Aeras, IDT Biologika form a strategic partnership with acquisition of Aeras's manufacturing facility." News release, June 23. www.prnewswire.com/news/aeras.

———. 2014. "AnnualReport." www.aeras.org/annualreport2014.

———. 2012a. "Award to Aeras boosts historic hunt for new vaccines against TB as drug-resistant strains proliferate." News release, March 15. www.aeras.org/pressreleases/award-to-aeras-boosts-historic-hunt-for-new-vaccines-against-tb-as-drug-res.

———. 2012b. "Aeras and CNBG sign agreement on tuberculosis vaccine R&D." News release, January 10. www.aeras.org/pressreleases/aeras-and-cnbg-sign-agreement-on-tuberculosis-vaccine-rd.

Akrong, Lloyd, K. Horstman, and D. Arhinful. 2014. "Informed consent and knowledge translation: perspectives on clinical trials from a Ghanaian community." In N. Engel, I. Van Hoyweghen, and A. Krumeich, eds., *Making Global Health Care Innovation Work: Standardization and Localization*, 17–40. New York: Palgrave Macmillan.

Apple, Rima. 1989. "Patenting university research: Harry Steenbock and the Wisconsin Alumni Research Foundation." *Isis* 80:375–94.

Arno, P., K. Bonuck, and M. Davis. 1995. "Rare diseases, drug development, and AIDS: the impact of the Orphan Drug Act." *Milbank Quarterly* 73, no. 2:231–52.

Balasegaram, Manica. 2014. "A novel solution for TB R&D." Session on Tuberculosis R&D Funding, 45th Union World Conference on Lung Health, Barcelona, Spain, October 31.

Barry, Andrew. 2005. "Pharmaceutical matters: the invention of informed materials." *Theory, Culture, and Society* 22, no. 1:51–69.

Basilico, M., J. Weigel, A. Motgi, J. Bor, S. Keshavjee. 2013. "Health for all? Competing theories and geopolitics." In P. Farmer, J. Y. Kim, A. Kleinman, and M. Basilico, eds., *Reimagining Global Health: An Introduction*, 74–110. Berkeley: University of California Press.

Bensaude-Vincent, B., and I. Stengers. 1996. *A History of Chemistry.* Cambridge, MA: Harvard University Press.

Biehl, Joao. 2011. "When people come first: beyond technical and theoretical quick-fixes in global health." In R. Peet, P. Robbins, and M. Watts, eds., *Global Political Ecology*, 100–30. London: Routledge.

Biehl, Joao, and Adriana Petryna. 2014. "Peopling global health." *Saúde e Sociedade* 23, no. 2:376–89.

———. 2013. "Critical global health." In J. Biehl and A. Petryna, eds., *When People Come First: Critical Studies in Global Health*, 1–22. Princeton, NJ: Princeton University Press.

Bishop, Matthew, and Michael Green. 2008. *Philanthrocapitalism: How the Rich Can Save the World.* New York: Bloomsburg Publishing.

Blowfield, Michael, and Jedrzej George Frynas. 2005. "Setting new agendas: critical perspectives on corporate social responsibility in the developing world." *International Affairs* 81, no. 3:499–513.

Brennan, M., and J. Thole. 2012. "Tuberculosis vaccines: a strategic blueprint for the next decade." *Tuberculosis* 92S1:S6–S13.

Brigden, Grania. 2011. "Capreomycin shortage: symptom of a bigger problem in multidrug-resistant tuberculosis." *PlosBlogs*, November 16.

Broadbent, Alex. 2011. "Defining neglected disease." *BioSocieties* 6, no. 1:51–70.

Bud, Robert. 2008. "Upheaval in the moral economy of science? Patenting, teamwork and the World War II experience of penicillin." *History and Technology* 24, no. 2:173–90.

Bull, Benedicte, and Desmond McNeill. 2007. *Development Issues in Global Governance: Public-Private Partnerships and Market Multilateralism.* London: Routledge/Taylor and Francis.

Buse, K., and A. Harmer. 2007. "Seven habits of highly effective global public–private health partnerships: practice and potential." *Social Science and Medicine* 64:259–71.

Buse, K., and G. Walt. 2000. "Global public–private partnerships: part I, a new development in health?" *Bulletin of the World Health Organization* 78:549–61.

Caminero, José. 2010. "Treatment of MDR-TB." Workshop on MDR-TB Management and Treatment, 41st Union World Conference on Lung Health, Berlin, Germany, November 12.

CDC (Centers for Disease Control and Prevention). 2010. "Treatment for TB disease: recommended regimens." www.cdc.gov/tb/topic/treatment/tbzdis ease.htm.

Chandhoke, Neera. 2012. "Who owes whom, why, and to what effect?" In S. Maffettone and A. S. Rathore, eds., *Global Justice: Critical Perspectives*, 143–62. London: Routledge.

Chaudhuri, Sudip. 2010. "R&D for development of new drugs for neglected diseases in India." *International Journal of Technology and Globalisation* 5, nos. 1–2:61–75.

Checkley, Anna, and Helen McShane. 2011. "Tuberculosis vaccines: progress and challenges." *Trends in Pharmacological Sciences* 32, no. 10:601–6.

Chen-Yuan, Chiang. 2010. "Mechanisms in the development of drug resistant TB." Workshop on MDR-TB Management and Treatment, 41st Union World Conference on Lung Health, Berlin, Germany, November 12.

Clayden, P., S. Collins, C. Daniels, M. Frick, M. Harrington, T. Horn, R. Jefferys, K. Kaplan, E. Lessem, L. McKenna, and T. Swan. 2014. *2014 HIV/HCV/TB Pipeline Report: Drugs, Diagnostics, Vaccines, Preventive Technologies, Research toward a Cure, and Immune-Based and Gene Therapies in Development.* Treatment Action Group i-base. www.pipelinereport.org/2014/TOC.

CPTR (Critical Path to TB Drug Regimens). 2016. "Regulatory authorities support first drug development tool, critical to advance TB R&D efforts." News release, March 19. www.cptrinitiative.org/2015/03/19/first-drug-development-tool -to-support-tb-regimen-development-supported-by-regulatory-authorities/.

———. 2015. "TB and HIV join together for combined community engagement forum." News release, December 21. www.cptrinitiative.org/2015/12/21/tb -hiv-join-together-for-combined-community-engagement-forum/.

———. 2010a. "FDA is easing way for drug cocktails." News release, March 18. www.cptrinitiative.org/2010/03/18/fda-is-easing-way-for-drug-cocktails/.

———. 2010b. "FDA, EMA, and global partners join forces to speed development of new TB drug combinations." News release, March 24. www.cptrini tiative.org/2010/10/28/stop-tb-partnership-launches-global-plan-to-stop -tb-2011-2015/.

Craddock, Susan. 2015. "Precarious connections: making therapeutic production happen for malaria and tuberculosis." *Social Science and Medicine* 129:36–43.

———. 2008. "Tuberculosis and the anxieties of containment." In H. Ali and R. Keil, eds., *Networked Disease: Emerging Infections in the Global City.* Blackwell Press Series on Studies in Urban Change. Oxford: Wiley-Blackwell.

Craddock, Susan, and Tamara Giles-Vernick. 2010. "Introduction." In T. Giles-Vernick and S. Craddock, eds., *Influenza and Public Health: Learning from Past Pandemics*, 1–21. London: Earthscan.

Crane, Johanna. 2014. Comments made during the Making African Capacity Workshop, Cambridge, England, June 14.

———. 2013. *Scrambling for Africa: AIDS, Expertise, and the Rise of American Global Health Science*. Ithaca, NY: Cornell University Press.

Cueto, Marcos. 2013. "A return to the magic bullet? Malaria and global health in the twenty-first century." In J. Biehl and A. Petryna, eds., *When People Come First: Critical Studies in Global Health*, 30–53. Princeton, NJ: Princeton University Press.

Daniels, Colleen. 2014. "Overcoming the challenges in TB R&D." Session on Tuberculosis R&D Funding, 45th Union World Conference on Lung Health, Barcelona, Spain, October 31.

DeBruin, D., J. Liaschenko, and A. Fisher. 2011. "How clinical trials really work: rethinking research ethics." *Kennedy Institute of Ethics Journal* 21, no. 2:121–39.

Diacon, Andreas, Lize vander Mewe, Christoph Lange, Alberto L. García-Basteiro, Esperança Sevene, and Lluís Ballell. 2016. "B-lactams against tuberculosis: new trick for an old dog?" *New England Journal of Medicine* July 23. DOI: 10.1056/NEJMc1513236.

Dowdy, David. 2014. "The potential impact of 3- and 4-month regimens: insights from modeling." Session on Clinical Trials for Drug Sensitive Tuberculosis, 45th Union World Conference on Lung Health, Barcelona, Spain, October 30.

Dumit, Joseph. 2012. *Drugs for Life: How Pharmaceutical Companies Define Our Health*. Durham, NC: Duke University Press.

Ecks, Stefan. 2008. "Global pharmaceutical markets and corporate citizenship: the case of Novartis's anti-cancer drug Glivec." *BioSocieties* 3, no. 2:165–81.

Emergent BioSolutions. 2009. "Oxford-Emergent Tuberculosis Consortium signs commercial license agreement with Vivalis to explore production of MVA85A TB vaccine candidate using EB66® cell line." News release, May 5. investors.emergentbiosolutions.com/phoenix.zhtml?c=202582&p=irol-newsArticle&ID=1284485.

Engel, N., I. Van Hoyweghen, and A. Krumeich, eds. 2014. *Making Global Health Care Innovation Work: Standardization and Localization*. New York: Palgrave Macmillan.

Evans, Tom. 2011. "New TB vaccines in clinical development." Presentation at the 42nd Union World Conference on Lung Health, Lille, France, October 28.

Farmer, Paul. 2004. *Pathologies of Power: Health, Human Rights, and the New War on the Poor*. Berkeley: University of California Press.

Farmer, P., J. Y. Kim, A. Kleinman, and M. Basilico, eds. 2013. *Reimagining Global Health: An Introduction*. Berkeley: University of California Press.

Farmer, P., M. Basilico, V. Kerry, M. Ballard, A. Becker, G. Bukhman, O. Dahl, A. Ellner, L. Ivers, D. Jones, J. Meara, J. Mukherjee, A. Sievers, and A. Yamamoto. 2013. "Global health priorities for the early twenty-first century." In P. Farmer, J. Y. Kim, A. Kleinman, and M. Basilico, eds., *Reimagining Global Health: An Introduction*, 302–39. Berkeley: University of California Press.

Fassin, Didier. 2013. "That obscure object of global health." In M. Inhorn and

E. Wentzell, eds., *Medical Anthropology at the Crossroads: Histories, Activisms, and Futures*, 95–115. Durham, NC: Duke University Press.

———. 2012. *Humanitarian Reason: A Moral History of the Present.* Berkeley: University of California Press.

Feinstein, C. H. 2005. *An Economic History of South Africa: Conquest, Discrimination, and Development.* Cambridge: Cambridge University Press.

Ferguson, James. 2010. "The uses of neoliberalism." *Antipode* 41:166–84.

Firestone, Raymond. 2011. "Lessons from 54 years of pharmaceutical research." *Nature Reviews: Drug Discovery* 10:963.

Fisher, Jill. 2008. *Medical Research for Hire: The Political Economy of Pharmaceutical Clinical Trials.* New Brunswick, NJ: Rutgers University Press.

———. 2007. "Coming soon to a physician near you: medical neoliberalism and pharmaceutical clinical trials." *Harvard Health Policy Review* 8, no. 1:61–70.

Fletcher, Helen, Margaret A. Snowden, Bernard Landry, Wasima Rida, Iman Satti, Stephanie A. Harris, Magali Matsumiya, Rachel Tanner, Matthew K. O'Shea, Veerabadran Dheenadhayalan, Leah Bogardus, Lisa Stockdale, Leanne Marsay, Agnieszka Chomka, Rachel Harrington-Kandt, Zita-Rose Manjaly-Thomas, Vivek Naranbhai, Elena Stylianou, Fatoumatta Darboe, Adam Penn-Nicholson, Elisa Nemes, Mark Hatherill, Gregory Hussey, Hassan Mahomed, Michele Tameris, J. Bruce McClain, Thomas G. Evans, Willem A. Hanekom, Thomas J. Scriba, and Helen McShane. 2016. "T-cell activation is an immune correlate of risk in BCG vaccinated infants." *Nature Communications* 7, May 6. DOI: 10.1038/ncomms11290.

Frick, Mike. 2015. "The tuberculosis vaccines pipeline: a new path to the same destination?" *2015 HIV/HCV/TB Pipeline Report*, Treatment Action Group i-base, www.pipelinereport.org/2015/tb-vaccines.

———. 2014. "The tuberculosis vaccines pipeline." *2014 HIV/HCV/TB Pipeline Report*, Treatment Action Group i-base. www.pipelinereport.org/2014/tb-vaccine.

Frimpong-Mansoh, A. 2008. "Culture and voluntary informed consent in African health care systems." *Developing World Bioethics* 8, no. 2:104–14.

Gabriel, Joseph. 2014. *Medical Monopoly: Intellectual Property Rights and the Origins of the Modern Pharmaceutical Industry.* Chicago: University of Chicago Press.

Gagneux, Sebastien, and Peter Small. 2007. "Global phylogeography of *Mycobacterium tuberculosis* and implications for tuberculosis product development." *Lancet Infectious Diseases* 7:328–37.

Galambos, Louis, and Jeffrey Sturchio. 1998. "Pharmaceutical firms and the transition to biotechnology: a study in strategic innovation." *Business History Review* 72, no. 2:250–78.

GAO (Government Accounting Office). 2006. "New drug development: science, business, regulatory, and intellectual property issues cited as hampering drug development efforts." GAO-07-49. www.gao.gov.

Gaudillière, Jean-Paul. 2008. "Professional or industrial order? Patents, biological drugs, and pharmaceutical capitalism in early twentieth century Germany." *History and Technology* 24, no. 2:107–33.

Geissler, W., A. Kelly, B. Imoukhuede, and R. Pool. 2008. "'He is now like a brother, I can even give him some blood': Relational ethics and material exchanges in a malaria vaccine 'trial community' in the Gambia." *Social Science and Medicine* 67:696–707.

Gikonyo, C., P. Bejon, V. Marsh, and S. Molyneux. 2008. "Taking social relationships seriously: Lessons learned from the informed consent practices of a vaccine trial on the Kenyan coast." *Social Science and Medicine* 67:708–20.

Gilpin, Christopher. 2011. "WHO update on GeneXpert MTB/RIF rollout." FIND workshop on New Diagnostics, 42nd Union World Conference on Lung Health, Lille, France, October 27.

Glickman, S., J. McHutchison, E. Peterson, C. Cairns, R. Harrington, R. Califf, and K. Schulman. 2009. "Ethical and scientific implications of the globalization of clinical research." *New England Journal of Medicine* 360, no. 8:816–23.

Global Fund to Fight AIDS, TB, and Malaria. 2015. Grant Overview. www.theglobalfund.org.

Goozner, Merrill. 2005. *The $800 Million Pill: The Truth Behind the Cost of New Drugs.* Berkeley: University of California Press.

Graves, Andrew, and David Hokey. 2011. "Tuberculosis vaccines: review of current development trends and future challenges." *Bioterrorism and Biodefense* S1:009.

Greene, J., M. Basilico, H. Kim, and P. Farmer. 2013. "Colonial medicine and its legacies." In P. Farmer, J. Y. Kim, A. Kleinman, and M. Basilico, eds., *Reimagining Global Health: An Introduction,* 33–73. Berkeley: University of California Press.

Hacking, Ian. 1995. *Rewriting the Soul: Multiple Personality and the Sciences of Memory.* Princeton, NJ: Princeton University Press.

Hamilton, Carol. 2013. "Engaging communities in research design." Workshop on Community Engagement, 44th Union World Conference on Lung Health, Paris, France, October 31.

Hanif, S., and L. Garcia-Contreras. 2012. "Pharmaceutical aerosols for the treatment and prevention of tuberculosis." *Frontiers in Cellular Infection Microbiology* 2:118.

Hayden, Cori. 2007. "Taking as giving: bioscience, exchange, and the politics of benefits-sharing." *Social Studies of Science* 37:729–758.

Healy, David. 2006. "The new medical oekimune." In Adriana Petryna, Andrew Lakoff, and Arthur Kleinman, eds., *Global Pharmaceuticals: Ethics, Markets, Practices,* 61–84. Duke University Press.

Herrling, P. 2007. "Patent sense." *Nature* 449, no. 13:174–75.

Heywood, M. 2002. "Drug access, patents, and global health: 'chaffed and waxed sufficient.'" *Third World Quarterly* 32, no. 2:217–31.

Horrobin, David. 2000. "Innovation in the pharmaceutical industry." *Journal of the Royal Society of Medicine* 92:341–45.

Hughes, Bethan. 2008. "2007 FDA drug approvals: a year of flux." *Nature Reviews: Drug Discovery* 7:107.

Institute for Health Metrics and Evaluation. 2014. "Financing Global Health." vizhub.healthdata.org.

Jasanoff, Sheila. 2006. "Biotechnology and empire: the global power of seeds and science." *Osiris* 21:273–92.

Jenkins, Rhys. 2005. "Globalization, corporate social responsibility and poverty." *International Affairs* 81, no. 3:525–40.

Jeong, Yeonbo. 2013. "'Leftover' embryos and ova for research: contested meanings of waste, body, and national development." *Korean Women's Studies* 29, no. 1:1–35.

Kaddar, Miloud. 2010. "Global Vaccine Market Features and Trends." World Health Organization. www.who.int/immunization/programmes_systems/procurement/market/world_vaccine_market_trends.pdf.

Kahn, Jonathan. 2012. *Race in a Bottle: The Story of BiDil and Racialized Medicine in a Post-Genomic Age*. Columbia University Press.

Kalipeni, E., S. Craddock, J. Oppong, and J. Ghosh, eds. 1994. *HIV and AIDS in Africa: Beyond Epidemiology*. Blackwell.

Koplan, J. P., T. C. Bond, M. H. Merson, K. S. Reddy, M. H. Rodriguez, N. K. Sewankambo, and J. N. Wasserheit. 2009. "Towards a common definition of global health." *The Lancet* 373, no. 9679:1993–95.

Katz, Michael L., Janusz A. Ordover, Franklin Fisher, and Richard Schmalensee. 1990. "R and D cooperation and competition." *Brookings Papers on Economic Activity: Microeconomics*, 137–203.

Kearns, G., and S. Reid-Henry. 2009. "Vital geographies: life, luck, and the human condition." *Annals of the Association of American Geographers* 99, no. 3:554–74.

Kelly, Ann, and Uli Beisel. 2011. "Neglected malarias: the frontlines and back alleys of global health." *BioSocieties* 6, no. 1:71–87.

Keshavjee, Salmaan. 2010. "Programmatic issues and barriers in implementing MDR-TB programs." Workshop on MDR-TB Management and Treatment, 41st Union World Conference on Lung Health, Berlin, Germany, November 12.

Keshavjee, Salmaan, and Paul Farmer. 2010. "Time to put boots on the ground: making universal access to MDR-TB treatment a reality." *International Journal of Tuberculosis and Lung Disease* 14, no. 10:1222.

Kesselheim, Aaron. 2011. "An empirical review of major legislation affecting drug development: past experiences, effects, and unintended consequences." *Milbank Quarterly* 89, no. 3:450–502.

Koplan, J., T. C. Bond, M. Merson, K. S. Reddy, M. H. Rodriguez, N. K. Sewankambo, and J. N. Wasserheit. 2009. "Towards a common definition of global health." *The Lancet* 373, no. 9679:1993–95.

Kuaban, Christopher. 2012. "Twelve-month standardized MDR-TB regimen: experience in Cameroon." Session on Advances in the Treatment of MDR-TB, 43rd Union World Conference on Lung Health, Kuala Lumpur, Malaysia, November 16.

———. 2011. "Preliminary results of 12-month standardized treatment for MDR-TB patients in Cameroon." Presentation at the 42nd Union World Conference on Lung Health, Lille, France, October 29.

Labonte, Ronald. 2001. "Liberalisation, health and the World Trade Organisation." *Journal of Epidemiology and Community Health* 55, no. 9:620–21.

Lairumbi, G. M., S. Molyneux, R. Snow, K. Marsh, N. Peshu, and M. English. 2008. "Promoting the social value of research in Kenya: Examining the practical aspects of collaborative partnerships using an ethical framework." *Social Science and Medicine* 67:734–47.

Lessem, Erika. 2014a. "Tuberculosis drug development hobbles forward." *2014 HIV/HCV/TB Pipeline Report*, Treatment Action Group i-base. www.pipelinereport.org/2014/tb-treatment.

———. 2014b. "An Activist's Guide to Delamanid." Treatment Action Group. www.treatmentactiongroup.org/tb /delamanid-factsheet.

Liese, Berhard, Mark Rosenberg, and Alexander Schratz. 2010. "Programmes, partnerships, and governance for elimination and control of neglected tropical diseases." *The Lancet* 375, no. 9708:67–77.

Light, Donald, and Joel Lexchin. 2012. "Pharmaceutical research and development: what do we get for all that money?" *British Medical Journal* 344:e4348.

Light, Donald, and Rebecca Warburton. 2011. "Demythologizing the high costs of pharmaceutical research." *BioSocieties* 6, no. 1:34–50.

Lockhart, Steve. 2013. Commentary at the Global TB Vaccines Trial, Cape Town, South Africa, March 26.

Ma, Zhenkun, Christian Lienhardt, Helen McIlleron, Andrew Nunn, and Xiexiu Wang. 2010. "Global tuberculosis drug pipeline: the need and the reality." *The Lancet* 375, no. 9731:2100–9.

MacPhail, Theresa. 2014. *The Viral Network: A Pathography of the H1N1 Influenza Pandemic.* Ithaca, NY: Cornell University Press.

Mahomed, H., R. Ehrlich, T. Hawkridge, M. Hatherill, L. Geiter, F. Kafaar, D. Abrahams, H. Mulenga, M. Tameris, H. Geldenhuys, W. Hanekom, S. Verver, and G. Hussey. 2013. "TB incidence in an adolescent cohort in South Africa." *PloS One* 8, no. 3:e59652.

Mahomed, H., T. Hawkridge, S. Verver, D. Abrahams, L. Geiter, M. Hatherill, R. Ehrlich, W. Hanekom, and G. Hussey. 2011. "The tuberculin skin test versus QuantiFERON TB Gold® in predicting tuberculosis disease in an adolescent cohort study in South Africa." *PloS One* 6, no. 3:e17934.

Marks, Harry M. 1997. *The Progress of Experiment: Science and Therapeutic Reform in the United States, 1900–1990.* Cambridge: Cambridge University Press.

Mbali, Mandisa. 2013. *South African AIDS Activism and Global Health Politics.* Basingstoke: Palgrave MacMillan.

McGoey, Linsey, Julian Reiss, and Ayo Wahlberg. 2011. "The global health complex." *BioSocieties* 6, no. 1:1–9.

McIlleron, H., P. Wash, A. Burger, P. Folb, and P. Smith. 2002. "Widespread distribution of a single drug rifampicin formulation of inferior bioavailability in South Africa." *International Journal of Tuberculosis and Lung Disease* 6, no. 4:356–61.

McKenna, Lindsay. 2015. "Momentum in the pediatric tuberculosis treatment pipeline." *2015 HIV/HCV/TB Pipeline Report.* Treatment Action Group i-Base. www.pipelinereport.org/2015/tb-pediatrics.

McKeown, Thomas. 1979. *The Role of Medicine: Dream, Mirage, or Nemesis?* Princeton, NJ: Princeton University Press.

McMillen, Christian. 2015. *Discovering Tuberculosis: A Global History 1900 to the Present.* New Haven, CT: Yale University Press.

Merry, Sally. 2011. "Measuring the world: indicators, human rights, and global governance." *Current Anthropology* 52, no. 3:S83–S95.

Messac, Luke, and Krishna Prabhu. 2013. "Redefining the possible: the global AIDS response." In P. Farmer, J. Y. Kim, A. Kleinman, and M. Basilico, eds., *Reimagining Global Health: An Introduction*, 111–32. Berkeley: University of California Press.

Millennium Project. 2006. "Millennium Development Goals: goals, targets, and indicators." www.unmillenniumproject.org.

Miller, T., and M. Boulton. 2007. "Changing constructions of informed consent: qualitative research and complex social worlds." *Social Science and Medicine* 65:2199–2211.

Mitchell, Timothy. 2000. "Introduction." In Timothy Mitchell, ed., *Questions of Modernity*, xi–xxvii. Minneapolis: University of Minnesota Press.

Mitnick, C., K. Castro, M. Harrington, L. Sacks, and W. Burman. 2007. "Randomized trials to optimize treatment of multidrug-resistant tuberculosis." *PloS Medicine* 4, no. 11:1–5.

Mol, Annemarie. 2002. *The Body Multiple: Ontology in Medical Practice.* Durham, NC: Duke University Press.

Moon, Suerie. 2014. "Demonstration financing: considerations for a pilot pooled International Fund for R&D." Drugs for Neglected Diseases Initiative, www.dndi.org/2014/advocacy/pilot-pooled-rd-fund.

Moran, Mary. 2005. "A breakthrough in R & D for neglected diseases: new ways to get the drugs we need." *Plos Medicine* 2, no. 9:e302.

Motsoaledi, Aaron. 2014. "Developing the global plan to stop TB, 2016–2020." Panel at the 45th Union World Conference on Lung Health, Barcelona, Spain, October 28.

Mowery, David, Richard Nelson, Bhaven Sampat, and Arvids Ziedonis. 2001.

"The growth of patenting and licensing by U.S universities: an assessment of the effects of the Bayh-Dole act of 1980." *Research Policy* 30:99–119.

MSF (Médecins Sans Frontières). 2011. "Access to lifesaving generic medicines threatened by US trade pact." Press release, September 7. www.doctorswith outborders.org/news-stories/press-release/access-lifesaving-generic -medicines-threatened-us-trade-pact.

———. 2009. "Problems of supply and availability for MDR TB drugs." www .msfaccess.org/main/tuberculosis/msf-and-tb.

———. 2003. "Doha derailed: a progress report on TRIPS and access to medicines." Médecins Sans Frontières briefing for the 5th WTO Ministerial Conference, Cancun, October 20.

Munos, Bernard. 2009. "Lessons from 60 years of innovation." *Nature Reviews: Drug Discovery* 8:959–68.

MVI (Malaria Vaccine Initiative). 2015. "Malaria vaccine candidate has demonstrated efficacy over 3–4 years of follow-up." www.malariavaccine.org/news -events/news/malaria-vaccine-candidate-has-demonstrated-efficacy-over -3-4-years-follow.

Nathan, Carl. 2007. "Aligning pharmaceutical innovation with medical need." *Nature Medicine* 13:304–8.

Newell, Peter. 2005. "Citizenship, accountability and community: limits of the CSR agenda." *International Affairs* 81, no. 3:541–57.

Newton, P., P. Tabernero, P. Dwivedi, M. Culzoni, M. Monge, I. Swamidoss, D. Milenhall, M. Green, R. Jahnke, M. dos Santos de Oliveira, J. Simao, N. White, and F. Fernandez. 2014. "Falsified medicines in Africa: all talk, no action." *The Lancet Global Health* 2, no. 9:e509–e510.

Nightingale, Paul. 2010. "Multidrug-resistant tuberculosis: narratives of security, global health care and structural violence." In Sarah Dry and Melissa Leach, eds., *Epidemics: Science, Governance, and Social Justice*, 165–88. London: Earthscan.

NSF (National Science Foundation). 2010. "Science and engineering indicators 2010, Chapter 5: Academic research and development." wayback.archive-it .org/5902/20160210151754/http://www.nsf.gov/statistics/seind10/.

Nunn, Andrew. 2010. "Defining endpoints in TB clinical trials." Presentation at the 41st Union World Conference on Lung Health, Berlin, Germany, November 14.

Ong, Aihwa. 2010. "Introduction: an analytics of biotechnology and ethics at multiple scales." In Aihwa Ong and Nancy Chen, eds., *Asian Biotech: Ethics and Communities of Fate*, 1–51. Durham, NC: Duke University Press.

———. 2005. "Ecologies of expertise: assembling flows." In A. Ong and S. Collier, eds., *Global Assemblages: Technology, Politics, and Ethics as Anthropological Problems*, 337–53. Malden, MA: Blackwell.

Ong, Aihwa, and Nancy Chen, eds. 2010. *Asian Biotech: Ethics and Communities of Fate*. Durham, NC: Duke University Press.

Oppenheimer, Gerald. 1988. "In the eye of the storm: the epidemiological construction of AIDS." In E. Fee and D. Fox, eds., *AIDS: The Burdens of History*, 267–300. Berkeley: University of California Press.

Packard, Randall. 2011. *The Making of a Tropical Disease: A Short History of Malaria*. Baltimore: Johns Hopkins University Press.

———. 1989. *White Plague, Black Labor: Tuberculosis and the Political Economy of Health and Disease in South Africa*. Berkeley: University of California Press.

Parry, Bronwyn. 2004. *Trading the Genome: Investigating the Commodification of Bio-Information*. New York: Columbia University Press.

Paul, Steven, Daniel Mytelka, Christopher Dunwiddie, Charles Persinger, Bernard Munos, Stacy Lindborg, and Aaron Schacht. 2010. "How to improve R&D productivity: the pharmaceutical industry's grand challenge." *Nature Reviews: Drug Discovery* 9:203–14.

Peterson, Kristin. 2014. *Speculative Markets: Drug Circuits and Derivative Life in Nigeria*. Durham, NC: Duke University Press.

Petroski, Henry. 2006. *Success through Failure: The Paradox of Design*. Princeton, NJ: Princeton University Press.

Petryna, Adriana. 2009. *When Experiments Travel: Clinical Trials and the Global Search for Human Subjects*. Princeton, NJ: Princeton University Press.

Petryna, Adriana, Andrew Lakoff, and Arthur Kleinman, eds. 2006. *Global Pharmaceuticals: Ethics, Markets, Practices*. Durham, NC: Duke University Press.

Pogge, T., and A. Hollis. 2011. "Epilogue: new drugs for neglected diseases." *Cambridge Quarterly of Healthcare Ethics* 20, no. 2:329–34.

Prahalad, C. K., and S. Hart. 2002. "The fortune at the bottom of the pyramid." *Strategy and Business* 26:115.

Quirke, Viviane. 2007. *Collaboration in the Pharmaceutical Industry: Changing Relationships in Britain and France, 1935–1965*. London: Routledge.

Rai, Arti, and Rebecca Eisenberg. 2003. "Bayh-Dole reform and the progress of biomedicine." *Law and Contemporary Problems* 66:289–314.

Raviglione, M. C., and A. Pio. 2002. "Evolution of WHO policies for tuberculosis control, 1948–2001." *The Lancet* 359, no. 9308:775–80.

Redfield, Peter. 2013. *Life in Crisis: The Ethical Journey of Doctors Without Borders*. Berkeley: University of California Press.

Rhodes, John. 2013. *The End of Plagues: The Global Battle Against Infectious Disease*. New York: Palgrave Macmillan.

Rose, Nikolas. 2006. *The Politics of Life Itself: Biomedicine, Power, and Subjectivity in the 21st Century*. Princeton, NJ: Princeton University Press.

Sariola, S., and B. Simpson. 2011. "Theorising the 'human subject' in biomedical research: international clinical trials and bioethics discourses in contemporary Sri Lanka." *Social Science and Medicine* 73:515–21.

Schrecker, Ted, Audrey Chapman, Ronald Labonté, and Roberto de Vogli. 2010. "Advancing health equity in the global marketplace: how can human rights help?" *Social Science and Medicine* 71:1520–26.

Schroeder, Ingrid. 2009. "The evolution of a 'European mode' of patent governance: legislation on the patenting of biotechnology in the European Union and in Germany." In Jean-Paul Gaudillière, Daniel J. Kevles, and Hans-Jörg Rheinberger, eds., *Living Properties: Making Knowledge and Controlling Ownership in the History of Biology*. Berlin: Max-Planck-Institut Für Wissenschaftsgeschichte.

Slinn, Judy. 2008. "Patents and the UK pharmaceutical industry between 1945 and the 1970s." *History and Technology* 24, no. 2:191–205.

Sparke, Mat. 2014. "Health." In Roger Lee, Noel Castree, Rob Kitchin, Victoria Lawson, Anssi Paasi, Christopher Philo, Sarah Radcliffe, Susan Roberts, and Charles Withers, eds., *Sage Handbook of Human Geography*, 680–704. Los Angeles: Sage Publications.

Stadler, Jonathan, and Eirik Saethre. 2011. "Blockage and flow: intimate experiences of condoms and microbicides in a South African clinical trial." *Culture, Health, and Sexuality* 13, no. 1:31–44.

Stadler, Jonathan, Sinear Delany, and Mdu Mntambo. 2008. "Women's perceptions and experiences of HIV prevention trials in Soweto, South Africa." *Social Science and Medicine* 66:189–200.

Stoever, Kari, and Jelle Thole. 2013. "TB vaccine research and development: a business case for investment." www.aeras.org/pdf/TB_RD_Business_Case _Draft_3.pdf.

Stop TB Partnership. 2014a. "Gamechanger: USAID and Janssen Therapeutics announce US$30 million worth of free bedaquiline to treat drug-resistant TB." News release, December 12. www.stoptb.org/news/stories/2014/nw14 _083.asp.

———. 2014b. "BRICS Health Ministers make historic commitments in the fight against TB." News release, December 5. www.stoptb.org/news/stories/2014 /ns14_081.asp.

———. n.d. "The global plan to stop TB: Progress and financial requirements." www.stoptb.org/assets/documents/resources/factsheets.

Strathern, Marilyn. 2000. "Accountability . . . and ethnography." In M. Strathern, ed., *Audit Cultures: Anthropological Studies in Accountability, Ethics, and the Academy*, 279–304. London: Routledge.

Sunder Rajan, Kaushik. 2012. "Pharmaceutical crisis and questions of value: terrains and logics of global therapeutic politics." *South Atlantic Quarterly* 111, no. 2:321–46.

———. 2006. *Biocapital: The Constitution of Postgenomic Life*. Durham, NC: Duke University Press.

Tameris, Michele. 2014. "Drama sets the stage: adolescent TB vaccine trials." Session on All Hands on Deck: Communication Engagement and TB Programmes, 45th Union World Conference on Lung Health, Barcelona, Spain, October 30.

———. 2013. "Challenges in TB vaccine trials." Workshop on Community Engagement, 44th Union World Conference on Lung Health, Paris, France, October 31.

Tameris, M., M. Hatherill, H. Mahomed, and H. McShane. 2013. "Tuberculosis vaccine trials—authors' reply." *The Lancet* 381, no. 9885:2254.

TB Alliance (Global Alliance for Tuberculosis Drug Development). 2015. "Global Phase 3 'STAND' trial launched to test new tuberculosis drug regimen PaMZ to shorten, improve treatment." News release, March 17. www.tballiance .org/news/global-phase-3-stand-trial-launched-test-new-tuberculosis -drug-regimen-pamz-shorten-improve.

———. 2014a. "TB Alliance spins-out non-TB assets to TenNor Therapeutics." News release, March 11. www.tballiance.org/news/tb-alliance-spins-out -non-tb-assets-tennor-therapeutics.

———. 2014b. "TB Alliance grants Fosun Pharma rights to develop, market promising TB cure in China." News release, April 22. www.tballiance.org /news/tb-alliance-grants-fosun-pharma-rights-develop-market-prom ising-tb-cure-china.

———. 2014c. "Novartis provides drug candidate compounds to TB Alliance." News release, August 18. www.tballiance.org/news/novartis-provides-drug -candidate-compounds-tb-alliance.

———. 2014d. "PA-824 has a new generic name: Pretomanid." News release, October 20. www.tballiance.org/news/pa-824-has-new-generic-name-pre tomanid.

———. 2013. "TB Alliance licenses late-stage TB program to CSIR-OSDD." News release, March 19. www.tballiance.org/news/tb-alliance-licenses-late-stage -tb-program-csir-osdd.

———. 2011. "China pioneers international R&D center for global health." TB Alliance News Center, March 23. www.tballiance.org/news/china-pioneers -international-rd-center-global-health.

———. 2009. "What countries want: the value proposition of existing and new first-line regimens for drug-susceptible tuberculosis." August. www.tb alliance.org/downloads/publications/TBA_VPSreport_final_flat.pdf.

———. 2000. "Executive summary of the scientific blueprint for TB drug development." www.tballiance.org/downloads/publications/TBA_Scientific _Blueprint_Exec.pdf.

Temin, Peter. 1980. *Taking Your Medicine: Drug Regulation in the United States.* Cambridge, MA: Harvard University Press.

Tindana, P. O., N. Kass, and P. Akweongo. 2006. "The informed consent process in a rural African setting: a case study of the Kassena-Nankana district of northern Ghana." *IRB: Ethics and Human Research* 28, no. 3:1–6.

Tobbell, Dominique. 2012. "Knowledgeable relations: the building of a pharmaceutical research network." In *Pills, Power, and Policy: The Struggle for Drug Reform in Cold War America and its Consequences*, 13–36. Berkeley: University of California Press.

Tsing, Anna. 2004. *Friction: An Ethnography of Global Connection.* Princeton, NJ: Princeton University Press.

UNDP (United Nations Development Programme). 2009. Millennium Development Goals, South Africa: Goal 6, Combat HIV/AIDS, malaria, and other diseases. Geneva. www.za.undp.org/content/south_africa/en/home/post-2015/mdgoverview.html.

Upadhyay, Pramod. 2013. "Comment on TB vaccine trials." *The Lancet* 381, no. 9885:2253.

USPTO (U.S. Patent and Trademark Office). 2010. "General information concerning patents." www.uspto.gov/patents-getting-started/general-information-concerning-patents.

Van Deun, Armand. 2012. "Nine-month standardized MDR-TB regimen in Bangladesh, an update." Session on Advances in the Treatment of MDR-TB, 43rd Union World Conference on Lung Health, Kuala Lumpur, Malaysia, November 16.

Weyer, Karin. 2012. "Diagnostics and drug resistance, WHO." New Diagnostics Working Group Meeting, 43rd Union World Conference on Lung Health, Kuala Lumpur, Malaysia, November 13.

WHO (World Health Organization). 2016. Malaria Fact sheet. www.who.int/mediacentre/factsheets/fs094/en.

———. 2015. *Global Tuberculosis Report.* 20th ed. Geneva: WHO.

———. 2009. *Tuberculosis Treatment Guidelines.* 4th ed. Geneva: WHO.

———. 2006a. *Public health, innovation and intellectual property rights: report of the Commission on Intellectual Property Rights, Innovation, and Public Health.* Geneva: WHO. www.who.int/intellectualproperty/documents/thereport/ENPublicHealthReport.pdf?ua=1.

———. 2006b. "Guidelines on Stability Evaluation of Vaccines." Geneva: WHO. www.who.int/biologicals/publications/trs/areas/vaccines/stability/Microsoft%20Word%20-%20BS%202049.Stability.final.09_Nov_06.pdf.

Whyte, Susan Reynolds, S. Van der Geest, and A. Hardon. 2002. *The Social Lives of Medicines.* Cambridge: Cambridge University Press.

Yanacopulos, Helen. 2011. "Combating transnational corporate corruption: Enhancing human rights and good governance." In Aurora Voiculescu and Helen Yanacopulos, eds., *The Business of Human Rights: An Evolving Agenda For Corporate Responsibility.* London: Zed Books.

Zunz, Olivier. 2012. *Philanthropy in America: A History.* Princeton, NJ: Princeton University Press.

Zvonareva, Olga, and Nora Engel. 2014. "Payments in clinical research: views and experiences of particants in South Africa." In N. Engel, I. Van Hoyweghen, and A. Krumeich, eds., *Making Global Health Care Innovation Work: Standardization and Localization.* New York: Palgrave Macmillan.

INDEX

bottom-of-the-pyramid (BOP) market model, 50
BPaZ, 39, 40
Brennan, Michael, 47
BRICS countries, 41–43, 50, 53–54, 134–36. *See also specific countries*
Broadbent, Alex, 17
Brundtland, Gro Harlem, 21, 31

CABs. *See* community advisory boards
capitalism, 5–6, 125
Carina's Choice, 104–5
Casenghi, Martina, 77, 84
Centers for Disease Control and Prevention (CDC), 8
Cepheid, 133
chemical libraries, 6, 77
China: licensing agreements, 118–19; PDP collaborations, 41–43, 51–56; tuberculosis rates, 51, 135
China National Biotech Group, 51
clinical trials: benefits, 113–16, 123; CABs in, 93, 104, 107, 108, 112, 123; categories of compounds in, 35–36; design parameters, 108–13, 124; distributive agency in, 116; efficacy of vaccines, 69–70, 78–79, 95; ethics of, 91–124; failure rates, 120–22; GCP in, 64–65, 96, 103, 104, 106, 108–9, 111; informed consent in, 92–93, 98, 106, 110–11, 122–23; and PDPs, 33–34, 39, 102, 115–16; phases, 7, 79; and political will, 102–3; and poverty, 91–92, 98–108, 122, 124; RCTs, 94–95, 112, 123; research ecologies, 116–20; risks, 91; sponsor obligations, 111–12; standardization and harmonization in, 47, 93, 95, 96, 123–24; training for, 113
collaborations and partnerships: with BRICS countries, 41–43, 50, 53–54,

134–36; halo effect, 50; of PDPs, 6, 10, 32–33, 35–40, 48–56, 59–60, 74, 86, 89, 118; university–industry, 11–14, 31, 48; on value, 49, 51, 76–77. *See also* product development partnerships
Combined Community Engagement Forum, 112
community advisory boards (CABs), 93, 104, 107, 108, 112, 123
Connolly, Jim, 43, 49
corporate social responsibility (CSR), 22–23, 49–50, 57, 77, 89
Council of Scientific and Industrial Research (CSIR), 118–19
Court of Appeals for the Federal Circuit, 13
CPTR. *See* Critical Path to TB Drug Regimens
Critical Path Institute, 82
Critical Path to TB Drug Regimens (CPTR), 82–85, 87, 88
CSIR. *See* Council of Scientific and Industrial Research
CSR. *See* corporate social responsibility

Day, Cheryl, 81, 88
DDW. *See* Drugs for Developing World (DDW) facility
delamanid, 35, 86, 114
Diamond vs. Chakrabarty, 13
diarylquinolines, 35–36
Directly Observed Therapy, Short-course (DOTS), 8, 100
DNDi. *See* Drugs for Neglected Diseases initiative
Doctors Without Borders. *See* Médecins San Frontières
Doha Declaration (2001), 16
DOTS. *See* Directly Observed Therapy, Short-course
drug resistance, 8–9

34–39, 44, 47–48, 79–80, 88, 121–22; as neglected disease, 18–19, 22, 94; persistence of, 1–3, 9, 17, 21, 23, 88, 91–92, 99, 128; regimen recommendations/testing, 8, 81–87; and technologies, 25–26, 117–18, 127–28; transmission of, 3, 17, 70, 97, 103, 128; treatment, 1, 5, 6–7, 35, 70–71, 128. *See also* clinical trials; multidrug-resistant tuberculosis

Tuberculosis Vaccine Initiative (TBVI), 32, 46

UNICEF. *See* United Nations Children's Fund

Union World Conferences on Lung Health, 28, 111, 134

United Nations Children's Fund (UNICEF), 43, 69, 118, 130

United Nations Development Programme, 130

University Technology Transfer Offices, 14

U.S. Agency for International Development (USAID), 21, 132

Vaccine Alliance. *See* GAVI

Verver, Suzanne, 102–3

Voss, Gérald, 69, 125–26

Wellcome Trust, 45–46, 75, 78

WHO. *See* World Health Organization

WIPO. *See* World Intellectual Property Organization

Worcester, South Africa: clinical trials, 46, 93, 98–107, 115

World Bank, 16, 130

World Health Organization (WHO), 1, 2, 3, 16; on GeneXpert, 19; on international health, 19; on neglected diseases, 18; Special Programme for Research and Training in Tropical Diseases, 113, 130; Stop TB Partnership, 7, 37, 46; tuberculosis regimen recommendations, 8; on vaccine stability, 72

World Intellectual Property Organization (WIPO), 75

World Trade Organization (WTO), 18

WTO. *See* World Trade Organization

XDR-TB. *See* extensively drug-resistant tuberculosis

Zambia: clinical trials, 46, 97

SUSAN CRADDOCK is professor in the gender, women, and sexuality studies department and the Institute for Global Studies at the University of Minnesota. She is author of *City of Plagues: Disease, Poverty, and Deviance in San Francisco* (Minnesota, 2000) and coeditor of *HIV and AIDS in Africa: Beyond Epidemiology* and *Influenza and Public Health: Learning from Past Pandemics.*